The Athletic Mom-To-Be

Training Your Way Into
Pregnancy and Motherhood

Jennifer Faraone & Dr. Carol Ann Weis

authorHOUSE®

AuthorHouse™
1663 Liberty Drive
Bloomington, IN 47403
www.authorhouse.com
Phone: 1-800-839-8640

Photographs by:
Shannon Ross
Brian Reiser

Edited by:
Janet Cocklin, Always Get It Write

Published by AuthorHouse   04/30/2015

ISBN: 978-1-4969-6150-1 (sc)
ISBN: 978-1-4969-6177-8 (hc)
ISBN: 978-1-4969-6149-5 (e)

Library of Congress Control Number: 2015900035

Certain stock imagery © Shutterstock

Print information available on the last page.

This book is printed on acid-free paper.

This book is for educational purposes and is intended for the athlete who is thinking about getting pregnant, is experiencing a healthy and non-complicated pregnancy, and/or has recently given birth. It does not replace the importance of seeing your health care providers regularly and reviewing your exercise goals and regime with them.

Contents

To Steve - without you, this book would not have been possible.
To Sophia and Dominic – you are my reasons for writing this book.
Love mom (Jennifer)

To My Family - without your love and support I am not sure I would
have completed this project.
Love Carol Ann

Many fears exist regarding exercise for the pregnant active woman. One can seek and find multiple position statements and guidelines from reputed international organizations like the Canadian Academy of Sport and Exercise Medicine and the American College of Sport Medicine describing safe exercise participation in pregnancy. This can be a difficult endeavor.

Exercise is not only safe but also beneficial for pregnant athletes from the recreational to the elite competitor. In *"The Athletic Mom-To-Be"*, the authors present a comprehensive accumulation of detailed information for women who want to either start or continue exercising during their pregnancy. Information is presented in an easy to read conversational style separated in distinct sections covering many aspects of physical activity. The reader will note sections include personal comments from well-known international female athletes who have exercised and trained during their pregnancies. Health care professionals will find the information evidenced-based and includes comments from known researchers and practitioners in the field of exercise and medicine. All women who want to maintain or improve their healthy lifestyle when they get the great news they are pregnant should explore this book.

Dr. Richard Goudie, MD, BSc, CCFP Dip Sports Medicine
President, Canadian Academy of Sport and Exercise Medicine, 2015

In my experience in interprofessional practice with leading spine specialty surgeons, each year at least one training session was devoted to dispelling medical myths that become bound to common practice. In their book *"The Athletic Mom-To-Be"*, Jennifer Faraone and Dr. Carol Ann Weis have assembled a guide through the maze of information and disinformation surrounding the athletic life style for women anticipating motherhood. Based on the relevant scientific literature and real world experience, they provide clear guidance for each person to consider their own baseline health, environment, nutrition, attitudes, beliefs and exercise habits. Advising and caring for one person effectively takes work. Managing two interdependent individuals may be more complex but should not be overwhelming in most cases. Congratulations to the authors on a readable and informative shepherding of moms, spouses and their coaches through personal decisions to improve their own health and happiness.

John J. Triano, DC, PhD, FCCS(C)
Professor, Research Canadian Memorial Chiropractic College, Toronto,
Associate Professor, Rehabilitation Sciences, McMaster University, Hamilton

FOREWORD

Kudos to Faraone and Weis for writing the answers to our questions, the solutions to our challenges and most importantly, the exercises that we can live by!

Pregnancy is such an important stage of any woman's life as it transitions her to motherhood, slowly but surely, with our bodies teaching us how to nurture ourselves and our young. Yet, despite centuries of observation of pregnancy, study of anatomy and examination of physiology, we truly are only beginning to appreciate the power of exercise during pregnancy. The evidence is clear, in a low risk pregnancy; exercise will help our mood, stabilize our blood sugar and condition our muscles. We are even learning that in high risk pregnancies, some movement is better than none. The days of shunning the sporty "mom-to-be" have been replaced by a social consciousness that healthy exercise is essential for healthy pregnancies.

Faraone and Weis have logically and scientifically provided a step-wise approach to incorporating training and exercise into the stages of pregnancy. They foster a philosophy of self-pacing, self-respect and thoughtful reflection. This is so important as it is the basis of using knowledge to create the tools for self-management. Today, more than ever, we need to engage and empower the consumer, the patient, the person as an active participant in their own health care plan. If one is engaged, they will be motivated and with motivation comes further engagement and then exercise becomes a self-fulfilling prophecy. However, the real hidden gem is the fact that mothers and fathers who are active have children who are active and then we start to change the health of future generations.

Readers will find that they journey through just enough anatomy to understand the core muscles, the pelvic girdle and cross training techniques. Practical advice, formulas and testimonials build a strong foundation based on current research and evidence that can be trusted. Every last detail is easy to read and supported by even more good information in the Appendices.

As a sport and exercise physician and author of the Exercise and Pregnancy Guidelines for the Canadian Academy of Sport and Exercise Medicine, I would like to congratulate the authors on a job well done and welcome this book as a solid pillar in the literature.

Dr. Julia Alleyne BHSc(PT) MD Dip Sport Med MScCH

Dr. Alleyne is the co-author of the 1998 and 2007 Exercise and Pregnancy Position Statement from the Canadian Academy of Sport Medicine and founder of the Exercise and Pregnancy Helpline at Women's College Hospital. She lectures and publishes internationally to inter-professional health care audiences on exercise prescription during and post pregnancy.

OUR STORY

Jennifer's Experience: So Many Questions
When I discovered that I was pregnant with my daughter Sophia, I immediately stopped training. More specifically, I immediately stopped training *hard!* As an experienced long-distance runner, I knew that it was relatively safe to run while pregnant. What I didn't know, however, was just how intense or long I could run. Like many other female athletes who become pregnant, I searched the internet, books and articles for answers. Unfortunately, I was quickly disappointed. The information was limited and did not provide the details that I needed. For example, I wanted to know:

- *Do I have to stop my training altogether now that I am pregnant?*
- *Will I put my baby or myself at risk if I continue with some harder workouts?*
- *Can I exercise more than the guidelines recommend?*

As I searched for answers to these questions, I grew more and more frustrated. Although I did come across some guidelines, I found them to be very conservative in nature and not necessarily taking into account the mom-to-be who may be in better shape than the general population. I found that different sources provided contrasting and, sometimes, conflicting answers. Furthermore, there was a strong focus on what *not* to do (with very little mention of the reasoning behind these restrictions) and not enough information on what *to do*. Talking to other athletic moms, I realized that I was not the only one searching for this type of information. In fact, their questions arose even before conception and continued into the postpartum period. For instance:

- *Does training affect my ability to conceive?*
- *How much training can I do while trying to get pregnant?*
- *How soon after giving birth can I start to exercise?*
- *How will I know when my body is ready to handle more vigorous workouts?*
- *Can I continue to breastfeed while training hard?*

More questions with limited answers!

The Search for Answers: Enter Dr. Carol Ann Weis

After numerous conversations with other athletic women and several health care providers who treated pregnant athletes, I realized that there was a need for a comprehensive book that would expand beyond the traditional guidelines and provide the answers to such questions. However, developing such a book would be no easy feat! I was then introduced to Dr. Carol Ann Weis, a chiropractor and personal trainer who specializes in exercise during pregnancy and conducts research at the Canadian Memorial Chiropractic College regarding low back pain and pregnancy. After working with a number of athletic moms-to-be, Carol Ann also believed there was a gap in the information. Desiring to provide her own patients with a valuable resource, Carol Ann knew that a book of this nature was not only warranted, but a necessity. With a shared passion and goals, a partnership was formed and the writing began.

Calling On The Experts

Although we were each bringing forward our personal knowledge, experience and passion to the writing, we knew that this was not enough. In order to provide the most relevant, accurate, and where feasible, scientific information, it was important that we tap into the following 3 sources:

- ***Research Experts*** – We summarized the latest research and presented it in an easy to read manner, including journal articles, books and websites. We also interviewed some of the most renowned researchers in the field of exercise and pregnancy to gain further insight and understanding.
- ***Clinical Experts*** - In addition to the more traditional health care providers that work with pregnant women, such as obstetricians

and family doctors, we also tapped into the road less travelled of complementary alternative medicine providers. These include midwives, osteopaths, naturopaths, massage therapists, chiropractors and physiotherapists.

- *The Athletic Moms* - In other words, those who have "been there, done that". In the spirit of collaboration and sisterhood out of which this project grew, we know that there is so much that we can learn and gain from one woman to another. Despite all of the valuable information that can be provided by the other 2 sources mentioned above, sometimes we just need to hear directly from someone that has gone through the experience herself.

Our Goals for This Book

One of our main goals in writing this book is to create a resource for athletic women of all fitness levels, as well as health care providers and exercise professionals. Furthermore, this book will reach *beyond* exercise and pregnancy, as we know that your questions do not end there. We strongly believe in the importance of providing you with a more holistic approach to your pregnancy, from pre-conception to postpartum. Pregnancy is not something that only impacts you physically; it affects you on all levels - including your body, mind and spirit. Therefore, our book addresses an entire range of other meaningful topics, such as:

- How to best prepare your body before getting pregnant.
- How to maintain a healthy body for exercising and training during the ongoing changes of pregnancy and birth.
- How to use your skills as an athlete to cope during your labour and delivery.
- How to adjust, not just physically but also mentally, to the change in pace during this 9-month period and beyond.
- How to know when your body is ready for increased level of exercise postpartum.
- How to establish a smart training program both during and after pregnancy.
- How to make sense of the common misconceptions regarding nutrition, breastfeeding and training.

Our final goal for this book is to make this information accessible to as many athletic women as possible, as we believe that anyone who puts their heart and mind into exercise is an athlete. The term "athlete" is not characterized by your performance level or the number of hours that you devote to training, but rather the choice that you make to be fit and active. So, regardless of whether you have been competing for years, recently started training or are just getting back into shape following the birth of your child, we believe that you will find no shortage of useful information in this book to guide you into pregnancy and motherhood. In fact, we guarantee that you will find yourself referring to this book time and time again!

Above All Else

Writing this book has been a wonderful experience for us. We sincerely hope that you find it to be informative and enjoyable, that it encourages you to be active before and during your pregnancy and that it will promote a safe, healthy and enjoyable return to training postpartum. That being said, and despite everything we know about the safety and the benefits of exercising while pregnant, if you simply do not feel comfortable or motivated to continue exercising during this time or if your health care provider has advised against it, it is important that you acknowledge and respect this decision. This should not be a time when you force yourself to get out the door and exercise or feel guilty about not training. Rather, it should be a time when you listen to what your mind, body and spirit require. Pregnancy and motherhood are treasured times to be embraced. If exercising can enhance these experiences, that's wonderful. If not, the road, the gym or the pool will be awaiting your return when the time is right for you and your new family!

THE GAME PLAN

Why is the information about exercise and pregnancy not always straightforward?
How do I make sense of all the information contained in this book?
Do I have to read the book from start to finish?

Why a Simple Answer is Not Always Available

Compared to 30 years ago, there is now much more information one can gather about exercise and pregnancy. For instance, many of the earlier concerns about the potential harmful effects of exercising during pregnancy have been put to rest. This increased knowledge is a result of the growing number of research studies and recommendations by experts in the field. In fact, there are a number of guidelines (as discussed in the chapter "To Train or Not To Train") regarding exercise during pregnancy that have been developed based on this research. That's the good news!

The not-so-good news is that there are still plenty of questions left unanswered. There remain many untapped areas of research regarding exercise and pregnancy, such as strength training and yoga. Furthermore, even less is known about other topics like the effects of *training* during pre-conception, pregnancy and postpartum or the role of alternative therapies for pregnant and postpartum athletes.

> ### The Difference Between Exercising and Training
>
> We differentiate between the terms exercising and training. *Training* is characterized by your commitment to some form of a plan that enables you to work toward a specific goal and may include larger volume and/or more intense activity. *Exercising* is used to describe your intention to incorporate physical activity in a less-scheduled manner, without a concrete goal or expectation.

So, how do you make sense of the available information or even the lack thereof? For starters, it is important to have a basic understanding of why there are limitations in research findings and how this curbs one's ability to make specific recommendations. There are multiple factors that may contribute to such limitations including:

- *Not all aspects of exercise during pregnancy can be examined.* Much research is based on studies involving animals pushed to exhaustion, often resulting in harmful effects for the animal and/or her fetus. For ethical reasons, this type of study would never be performed with pregnant women, therefore hindering our ability to draw conclusions.
- *Not all studies are created equal.* There are many types of studies, some of which provide stronger evidence and from which firm recommendations can be made. A study that is considered to produce the strongest results is known as a randomized control trial (RCT). Unfortunately, there is not an RCT for every aspect of exercise and pregnancy; reliance on other types of studies is required. For instance, case studies have a lot of clinical value and are frequently considered, even though they are considered a weaker source of evidence.
- *The use of poorly defined or inconsistent terminology.* Researchers, for example, may define the terms "light", "moderate" and "heavy" effort/intensity differently, making it harder to draw conclusions or compare findings.
- *The manner in which certain studies are performed.* Certain factors, such as a small number of participants or the lack of a comparison group, can limit the interpretation of the findings or how we are able to use their conclusions.

Not surprisingly, it may be difficult for many people to sort through and make sense of all of the available information – unless you have a scientific background or a PhD. That brings us back to this book's use of other equally important sources of information, including the research and clinical experts and the real life experiences of athletic moms.

Navigating this Book

Given the complexity of the research, the abundance of topics and the depth of information that can be explored, we wrote this book according to the 3 phases of your journey to motherhood:

- Pre-conception
- Pregnancy
- Postpartum

You do not necessarily have to read this book from start to finish, as we know that it may not be possible or practical due to lack of time and/or personal preference. Therefore, we wrote the book in such a way that you can pick it up at *any* point during your journey. For example, you can jump straight to the postpartum section if you have already given birth. For ease of reading, we have organized the book in the following manner:

- Each of the 3 phases is broken down into specific chapters, each focusing on a particular topic.
- Every chapter begins with a series of questions highlighting the information that will be addressed.
- Helpful sidebars appear in each chapter to further illustrate and reinforce the message we are trying to convey.
- A list of helpful resources and references appears at the back of the book.

Combined, we hope that these efforts will empower you to be proactive during your journey into pregnancy and motherhood, to help you understand your experiences as they happen and to prepare you for what's to come. So, read on and enjoy!

YOUR WARM UP

This book provides a wealth of information, so that you can make informed decisions about what is best for you and your baby as they relate to a variety of exercise and other meaningful topics that span the pre-conception, pregnancy and postpartum periods. This is not an easy task given that no two women or two pregnancies are the same. We hope to address this challenge by providing you with a "one-stop shop" that contains all of the relevant information at your fingertips.

However, that is only part of the equation of what makes this book a valuable resource. The other half comes from you, and more specifically, your ability to be honest with yourself with respect to your own pre-conceived ideas and expectations toward your upcoming pregnancy and journey into motherhood. We therefore encourage you to take a moment to reflect on the following questions:

- *What do I expect from myself with respect to training throughout my pregnancy and once I become a mom?*
- *What and where do these expectations stem from?*
- *Am I prepared to significantly decrease my training (or stop it all together) if need be?*
- *What questions do I have about additional topics such as breastfeeding, nutrition and labour?*
- *What type of information am I seeking from this book?*

Having this private conversation with yourself will not only help you better navigate this book, but it will also ensure that you are getting the answers you need. More importantly, this reflection will enable you to make your decisions with confidence, reassurance and ease.

PREPARING YOUR BODY FOR PREGNANCY

Chapter 1

TRAINING FOR CONCEPTION

Does being an athlete affect my ability to conceive?
Should I stop training if I'm trying to get pregnant?
What can I do to increase my chances of getting pregnant?

Exercise and Fertility at a Glance
Exercise and fertility is a topic that has its share of differing views, findings and generalizations. For instance, some physically active women experience significant difficulty in trying to conceive, whereas others become pregnant within their first couple of months of trying. Karen Cockburn, a Canadian Olympic trampolinist and mother of 1, tried for just several months when she became pregnant shortly after competing in the 2012 Summer Olympics. Fiona Whitby, a professional triathlete and mother of 1, tried for 7 years before finally conceiving.

Some health care providers and exercise professionals will initially advise women to cut back on their training, whereas others will encourage them to continue their training regime while attempting to become pregnant. Jenny Hadfield, endurance training coach and author, often recommends decreasing both the training volume and intensity. Hadfield also encourages women to look at other factors that may impact their fertility, such as their nutrition and stress levels. On the other hand, Dr. Clifford Librach, Director of the Create Fertility Centre and Associate Professor in the Department of Obstetrics and Gynecology at the University of Toronto, does not encourage his patients to discontinue their training regime at first, provided that they have regular periods. However, if they encounter difficulties conceiving or have absent or irregular periods, he suggests considering whether an excessive amount of training may be impacting their fertility.

Why do some women get pregnant right away and others do not? Why such differences in the approach and advice given by health care and exercise professionals? As illustrated by the length of this chapter, your fertility can be a complicated topic. Fortunately, the intent of this chapter is not to discuss all of the ABC's of fertility; rather we felt it more important to provide a basic overview of fertility and how it relates to your training.

Early Studies and Generalizations
Dr. James Clapp, author of *Exercising Through Your Pregnancy*, suggested that some of these concerns were partly due to the stereotypical thinking of some individuals, including medical professionals, when it came to the active woman and her fertility. Clapp proposed that some health care providers, for example, believed that active women experienced abnormal reproductive function as a result of being underweight, malnourished and highly stressed, both physically and emotionally. Clapp further suggested that such health care providers thought that these 3 factors would not only influence fertility, but potentially could also influence the course and outcome of pregnancy, such as low birth weight babies. He also believed that conclusions were often based on subjective, rather than objective findings and generalizations were quickly made. For example, the commonly held belief that athletic and underweight women will have difficulty getting pregnant arose from an eating disorder study stating that a woman's percentage of body fat needed to be between 18-21% to ensure normal menstruation and ovulation.

Wanting to dig deeper into the matter, Clapp and colleagues examined the exercise habits of 250 recreational athletes who were unable to conceive within 6 months and exercised 3-5 times per week for 20-60 minutes. They compared this group to a group of 250 women that did not exercise. No differences were found between the groups. This led Clapp and colleagues to suggest that most healthy women can exercise at a moderately hard to hard intensity without interfering with fertility. They further cautioned that there might be an exercise threshold level above which infertility may become a problem.

The Bottom Line

So the question becomes, *can you still continue to train, even at a greater intensity, while trying to get pregnant?* The short answer is "yes". Training does not necessarily mean that you will have difficulty getting pregnant. Plenty of women have conceived during their normal training season, intentionally or not. The more thorough answer to the question is – "it depends", as fertility is based on numerous and often inter-related factors that may vary from person to person. Such factors can include: age, illness, gynecological issues, hormonal abnormalities, nutritional deficiencies, excessive exercise, emotional or mental disturbances, and, of course, your partner's ability to produce sperm. Furthermore, the likelihood of conceiving is lowered when more than one factor is present.

In other words, training is just *one* of several factors that can affect your fertility. Given that some of these factors can be more prominent with athletes, such as a low body mass index (BMI) or nutritional deficiencies, it becomes increasingly important to look at the *complete* picture. Librach suggests looking at your difficulty to conceive as a puzzle. In order to get the complete picture, you need to figure out how all the pieces fit together. Furthermore, assuming that your inability to get pregnant is due entirely to your training, without considering other factors, could lead to an unnecessary delay in treatment.

Another consideration is that your medical doctor may not speak to you regarding your inability to have a child until you have been trying for some time, in many cases at least a year. For example, the American Society of Reproductive Medicine recommends that a woman aged 35 or under consults her health care provider only after she has been trying to conceive for more than 12 months. For women over the age of 35, this timeframe is shortened to 6 months. Remember, these are only guidelines, since there are many circumstances where waiting this long would not be advisable. Examples include: a lack of, or very infrequent

> **Start Shopping Around Now**
> If you are planning to train throughout your pregnancy, you may want to start giving consideration now to finding an obstetrician or midwife with the most up-to-date knowledge and experience working with athletes. This person should be comfortable with your decision to continue some form of training, as long as you are experiencing a healthy and non-complicated pregnancy. A shared understanding will help to facilitate an open dialogue with your provider, so that you will feel comfortable discussing all aspects of your training.

periods, history of a severe pelvic infection or sexually transmitted infection, previous pelvic surgery, a history of endometriosis, a partner who has testicular surgery or prior cancer treatments in either partner.

So, what should you do once you are ready to get pregnant? Stop training? Continue training? Run to the nearest fertility expert? Start thinking about the other potential factors? Before getting too overwhelmed, a simple, and perhaps logical first step is to learn about what you can do proactively to increase your chances of conceiving.

Understanding Your Fertility
There are certain risk factors and conditions, such as obesity and polycystic ovary syndrome, which may require you to seek the assistance of medical professionals and are beyond the scope of this book. However, many of you will not require such intervention, at least not initially, as a number of the factors that can affect fertility can be influenced by your actions. As such, we have simplified this topic by focusing on those factors that are likely most relevant to you as an athlete:

1. Low BMI
2. Inadequate calorie and/or nutritional intake
3. Variations in training
4. Excessive training
5. High stress and anxiety

Identifying which of these 5 factors, if any, could be affecting your ability to get pregnant may be tricky, as there is often overlap among them. As a result, some guesswork and a little bit of trial and error are usually required. Although each of these factors is unique and can affect your fertility in slightly different ways, they all share one common outcome: *their ability to cause irregular periods.* As such, it is important to pay attention to your menstrual cycle, as it can provide a sign when something is not working properly. "Your menstrual cycle acts as a gage - when there are changes to your menstrual cycle, including a lack of one, it is a sign that something is going on," explains Librach.

That is not to say that any of the 5 factors will definitely lead to irregular periods and infertility. Instead, they are simply a consideration that any of the 5 factors may have certain thresholds that, when reached, could potentially affect your menstrual cycle and subsequently your fertility. Furthermore, there may be other causes of irregular periods, emphasizing the importance of engaging your doctor in a dialogue early on. Finally, we are not recommending that you take action only if you experience irregular periods. On the contrary, we are suggesting that you take a hands-on approach and gain a better understanding of how each factor could potentially affect your fertility *before* it becomes a problem. Let's begin by providing a basic overview of your menstrual cycle followed by a brief explanation of the 5 factors.

Your Menstrual Cycle

The length of the menstrual cycle varies from woman to woman, cycle to cycle, year to year and decade to decade. However, most women of childbearing age report their cycle lasts for approximately 28 days. The menstrual cycle is split into 3 phases: follicular, ovulatory and luteal phase (Table 1.0).

The purpose of the menstrual cycle is simple; with the help of several fluctuating hormones, it readies an egg to be released into the fallopian tube with the hopes of meeting a sperm and becoming fertilized. It also prepares the lining of the uterus for the possible implantation of that egg. If no implantation occurs, the lining breaks down and is discharged. This discharge is referred to as menstruation, also known as your "period".

Table 1.0: Overview of the Menstrual Cycle

Phase	Purpose	Primary Hormones
Follicular	• Maturation of eggs	• Follicular Stimulating Hormone (FSH) • Estrogen
Ovulatory	• Release of the mature eggs into the fallopian tubes (ovulation occurs) • Occurs ~13 days prior to the start of your period	• Luteinizing Hormone (LH)
Luteal	• Preparation of uterine lining • Implantation of the fertilized egg (if conception occurs) or menstruation	• Progesterone

This is your menstrual cycle in a nutshell. The bottom line is that in order to get pregnant, you must be ovulating. But what happens if you do not ovulate?

A Not-So-Normal Menstrual Cycle
Simply having your period does not necessarily mean that you are ovulating. It is possible to have a period without ovulation and vice versa. Some signs that you are ovulating may include a noticeable change in your cervical mucus to an "egg white-like" consistency, a sharp pain around 14 days before the onset of your period and premenstrual symptoms called molimina (e.g. breast tenderness, bloating and mood changes). There are different types of menstrual disturbances that you may experience:

- Regular cycles with shortened luteal phase; progesterone production stops early
- Regular cycles with inadequate progesterone production
- Regular cycles with failure to develop and release an egg (anovulation)
- Irregular cycles but still ovulating
- Irregular cycles and anovulation (no ovulation)
- Absence of both menses and ovulation (amenorrhea)

Although in some cases you may not even notice anything abnormal with your menstrual cycle, it is important to realize that such disturbances could impact your fertility. How common are menstrual disturbances in athletes? It is interesting to note that menstrual disturbances were reported in 6-79% of women involved in all degrees of physical activity. Amenorrhea is more commonly found in elite athletes whose sport emphasizes thin physiques with low BMI, such as ballet and endurance running. Additional studies reported the following results:

- Roupas and Georgopoulos (2011) suggested that menstrual disorders occur in 24-26% of runners. Specifically, amenorrhea increased in US collegiate runners from 3-60% as the training distance increased from less than 13 km to more than 113 km per week.
- Marquez and Moinero (2013) stated that asymptomatic menstrual disorders, such as anovulation, are common and have

been reported to occur at least once every 3 months in 78% of runners with regular menstrual cycles.

- Redman and Loucks (2005) reported that the percentage of 425 female collegiate athletes who had not menstruated by age 16 (primary amenorrhea) was 7.4% overall and 22% in three aesthetic sports (cheerleading, diving and gymnastics).

Although the above results may sound a bit disheartening, do not let them discourage you. As stated at the beginning of this chapter, fertility is based on numerous and often inter-related factors, many of which you have the power to influence. As such, the remainder of this chapter will focus on the 5 factors that we believe are most applicable to the athletic woman: BMI, calorie and/or nutritional intake, variations in training, excessive training and stress and anxiety.

Low Body Mass Index

BMI is a commonly used tool to determine your relative health. It is based on your height and weight and is related to your percentage of body fat. The link between BMI and fertility is based on the idea that some of the hormones responsible for reproduction, such as estrogen, are stored in your body's fat layers; when you have a low percentage of body fat, you may produce a smaller amount of such hormones, disrupting your menstrual cycle and making it difficult to become pregnant. Conversely, having too much body fat may also disrupt the hormonal balance. In fact, researchers in the United States suggest that people who are obese and sedentary may experience greater infertility than those who are not. Librach explains "it is not just the amount of fat present, but the location or distribution of the fat that is very important. Fat around your internal body organs can have different effects on your hormones and can increase your chances of developing conditions such as diabetes and heart disease and menstrual disturbances."

According to Health Canada, the "normal" or "healthy" BMI range is between 18.5 and 24.9. As with most things, however, BMI is not an exact science and there are some exceptions. For instance, Health Canada states that the BMI classification may not be as applicable to certain adults, such as pregnant and lactating women, those who are highly muscular and those who have a very lean body build. Furthermore, this cause-and-effect relationship between low BMI and hormonal disruption does not affect everyone in the same way, nor does it mean that everyone

Looking Beyond BMI

Although BMI is often considered when discussing fertility, Dr. Clifford Librach, Director of the Create Fertility Centre suggests also looking at muscle mass, otherwise referred to as lean body mass. Why? "There is enough evidence to suggest that a low lean body mass will affect ovulation," explains Librach. He further explains that BMI (which is based on height and weight) can be misleading, as it does not take into account the fact that muscle weighs more than fat. Consider the following 2 individuals with the same height and weight and therefore, the same BMI: the muscular athletic woman and the non-athletic pear-shaped sedentary woman. Not only do both women look physically different, but their fertility may be different as well. The non-athletic woman probably has a higher fat to muscle ratio and may potentially have a harder time conceiving. This brings us back to our earlier point in which having too much fat tissue may affect the hormonal balance, which in turn may affect your ability to get pregnant.

with a low BMI will have difficulty conceiving. There are plenty of athletes with a low BMI who are still considered "fertile healthy" and are able to get pregnant.

As an athlete wanting to get pregnant, when should you pay more attention to your BMI? Dr. Barrett, a high-risk obstetrician at Sunnybrook Health Sciences Centre, explains that a low BMI becomes a problem only once it starts to affect the menstrual cycle and specifically, ovulation. He therefore suggests using your menstrual cycle as a starting point – if you period is normal and comes approximately every 28 days, there is a good chance that your BMI will not be a factor.

Inadequate Calorie and/or Nutritional Intake

Inadequate calorie and/or nutritional intake can potentially affect your menstrual cycle and fertility when any of the following conditions are met:

- Restricting the total number of calories ingested.
- Restricting certain food groups (e.g. carbohydrates or fat).
- Eating too many foods lacking adequate nutritional content.

In addition to the more obvious relationship between calories, nutrition and BMI, your diet can indirectly affect your fertility in more ways than one, explains Tara Postnikoff, Holistic Nutritionist and Personal Trainer. Postnikoff explains that it is not the diet itself that leads to infertility, but rather the consequences of not ingesting the right amount or type of calories and nutrients. For instance, restricting too many calories or certain foods can lead to depletion of key nutrients including calcium, iron, vitamin B and zinc, all of which can affect fertility. Furthermore, a low calorie intake can also affect certain hormones, such as elevating cortisol (otherwise known as the stress hormone) or decreasing certain sex hormones like progesterone, which in turn, can also affect your fertility.

What is Your Daily Calorie Intake?

As an athlete, you likely need to consume more calories than the average person, as your daily calorie requirement is influenced largely by your activity levels. If the standard daily guideline for the average adult woman is 1,800-2,200 calories per day, you can assume that your daily calorie intake will be higher based on the type and volume of your exercise. Consider the daily calorie intake of several professional athletes during race season:

- Deena Kastor (103 lbs.), Olympic medalist, marathoner: 4,000 calories
- Sarah Hammer (135 lbs.), World Champion Cyclist: 4,500 calories
- Cherry Haworth (300 lbs.), Olympic Weightlifter: 3,000-4,000 calories

There are formulas and professionals that can help you accurately determine your calorie intake. However, you should be aware of the signs that you are not consuming enough calories, which include:

- Losing weight or not putting on the recommended amount
- Low energy levels during the day
- Frequent illness
- A drop in your workout performance
- The inability to focus/concentrate or remember things
- Consistently feeling irritable or anxious throughout the day

As mentioned previously, there is also the "cumulative effect" that comes into play, such as the combination of inadequate calorie intake *and* intense exercise, which together may lead to menstrual irregularities. This happens when the nutritional intake does not balance the amount of energy spent while exercising. The body starts to think that it is in "starvation mode". When this happens, the body begins to slowly shut down areas that are deemed less critical for survival, including the reproductive system.

How do you know if you should be paying more attention to your diet? As with many of the other factors, it is hard to determine at first glance whether your nutrition could be affecting your fertility. A good starting point is to look at the caloric volume and the variety of food groups that you consume in a typical day, including what you eat before, during and after your workout. Consider the following:

- Are your caloric needs being met?
- Are you eating a well-balanced diet consisting of whole grains and complex carbohydrates, lean protein and good fats?
- Are you avoiding certain types of food?

Even if you believe that you eat fairly well, it is a smart idea to evaluate your diet prior to getting pregnant. Some specialists recommend starting to prepare the body 12 months in advance of pregnancy as a way of cleansing the body through better nutrition.

Variations in Training
Unless you are training excessively, many experts agree that it is not necessarily the *amount* of training that limits your ability to conceive but rather, a sudden and drastic *change* to your regular training schedule. This includes a significant and rapid increase in the quantity of training (i.e. the number of dedicated hours per week) or the quality or intensity of training (i.e. adding an additional speed workout each week). When such changes occur, your body may perceive them as a sudden stressor and send a message to your brain to stop or shorten your ovulation phase. "Your brain's hormonal control centres regress to a state that is similar to what they were like before puberty," explains Librach.

If and when you try to conceive, it is best to keep your training program fairly consistent in terms of quantity and quality. Alternatively, if you do want to mix up your training, try increasing just one aspect of training at a time, in small increments, no more than 10% per week. For instance, increase or decrease your weekly mileage by 5-10% while keeping the frequency and intensity of your workouts consistent.

Excessive Training
There does not exist a set of criteria that defines "excessive training". This is an individual factor that is often based on your previous training history as it relates to intensity, frequency and duration. Furthermore, the threshold for "excessive" training and at which point it can affect fertility, varies from one woman to the next. Although it is commonly suggested to decrease one's training when experiencing difficulty conceiving, it is

interesting to note that the studies concerning the amount of training and its impact on fertility seem to have varying results. For instance, some studies have found that vigorous exercise of 1 hour per day was not associated with infertility. In comparison, another study suggested that lean women who exercise vigorously more than 5 hours per week may improve their chances of becoming pregnant if they switch to a more moderate physical activity regime. As you can see, it can be difficult to quantify the exact threshold of exercise upon which fertility becomes compromised.

Given such differing results, it is increasingly important to rely on expert opinion. Librach, whose practice is comprised of 5-10% athletes, defines "excessive" exercise as "marathon type distance running or activities that are figure-dependent such as ice skating". It is perhaps equally important to keep in mind that the threshold for excessive exercise may be met sooner when paired with other factors, such as stress or a low BMI. Therefore, rather than focusing on what is "excessive" and wondering if this applies to you, try focusing on the other signs and symptoms that might give you an indication that your level of training needs to be scaled back. These may include:

- Constant fatigue
- Frequent injuries
- Elevated resting heart rate
- Irregular menstrual cycle

High Stress and Anxiety
There is an increasing body of evidence that stress and anxiety can also alter the timing of your ovulation phase. Stress and anxiety stems from many sources, including the more obvious day-to-day triggers like tight deadlines at work and financial concerns, to a more generalized anxiety featuring constant worrying. But did you know that your training could also be a source of stress? For instance, there may be times when your training regime itself may create anxiety, perhaps more so if you are committed to a particular training plan or are training for a specific event. If you respond "yes" to any of the following questions, it may be time to revisit and adjust your training plan:

- Is your stomach in knots prior to every workout?
- Do you feel that your program is too ambitious?

- Are you constantly tired and maybe even irritable during or after your workouts?
- Do you have difficulty finding the time to fit in all your workouts?
- Are you often injured?

On the flip side, exercising can also be a great way to relieve daily stress by providing you with the opportunity to clear your head, reflecting on whatever has been bothering you, or simply giving you the opportunity to just "tune out" from the world around you. Furthermore, exercise has the power to make you feel better. Given that the relationship between stress and your training can be both positive and negative, it is essential that your workouts function as a stress reliever rather than a stress generator.

Increasing Your Chances
Let us reinforce - you should not automatically assume that you will have difficulty conceiving solely because you are an athlete. That being said, there are certain steps that you can take to increase your chances of getting pregnant. An important first step is to learn more about the 5 factors that could potentially have an impact on your fertility and compare them to your current lifestyle. The second step is then to decide which factors, if any, will require additional consideration and possibly warrant some changes. For instance, the American College of Sports Medicine (ACSM) suggests that if your irregular period is as a result of excessive training, inadequate nutrition and a low BMI, you may be able to normalize your period by cutting back on your training by 10-15%, increasing your daily calorie intake and reaching your optimal weight.

How small of a change is big enough to make a difference? In their review of intense exercise on the female reproductive system, Warren and Perlroth (2001) suggested that either a weight gain of 1-2 kg (or 2.2-4.4 lbs.) or a 10% decrease in either exercise duration or intensity was enough to make a difference. Such small amounts are encouraging! Furthermore, you may be pleasantly surprised by how simple changes to your lifestyle, such as practicing daily meditation to better manage your stress or making positive changes to your diet, can positively influence your fertility.

Of special consideration is your age, since the quality and quantity of your eggs can become more of an issue around your mid 30's. In such a case, you may want to consider seeking medical assistance earlier. The same concept applies to your partner's sperm; do not hesitate in getting him checked out, as he is part of the puzzle Librach described earlier in the chapter.

Lastly, Librach lists the following signs of fertility issues that may warrant further medical assistance:

It May Not Be All You!

Although it is beyond the scope of this book, it is worthwhile to mention that any challenges trying to conceive could be related to your husband or partner's contribution. In fact, 40% of infertility cases are related to abnormal sperm, including a low sperm count or reduced motility. There are various causes for abnormal sperm, including training in warmer environments, frequent use of very hot baths or saunas, participating in contact sports and even spending a considerable amount of time cycling (not to mention wearing tight shorts). So, why not have him assessed by a health care provider, as well?

- Painful menses requiring pain relievers to function
- Menstrual pain that increases over time or is relieved by birth control pills
- Changes in your bowel and bladder function during menses
- Significant fatigue with menses
- A history of sexually transmitted infections, such as gonorrhoea or chlamydia
- A history of pelvic surgery or ruptured appendix
- Problems with excess body hair or acne
- Milky discharge from your nipples
- Issues with your thyroid

Summary

Despite what some people may think, you *can* continue to train while trying to get pregnant, at least initially. Although there are numerous factors that could affect your ability to get pregnant, the good news is that many of them are within your control. For starters, monitor your menstrual cycle for any irregularities, as this is could be a sign of potential fertility problems. To further increase your chances of conceiving, consider maintaining a healthy BMI of 18.5 or higher, paying attention to your calorie and nutritional intake, avoiding sudden and drastic changes to your training regime and if need be, cutting back on your workouts. In general, consider seeking medical assistance if you have been trying to conceive for 6 months to 1 year without success.

Chapter 2

GETTING YOURSELF
TO THE START LINE

I'm already fit ...won't my body be strong enough to handle my pregnancy?
What can I do to better prepare my body for the upcoming demands of
pregnancy?
How will this benefit me?

Your Pre-Conception Priorities
Although it may be more common to think about how to stay in shape
during pregnancy, less consideration is usually given to how you might
better prepare your body *ahead of time* for the upcoming physical
demands of pregnancy and labour. Being fit and physically strong prior
to getting pregnant is a benefit; however, these alone do not guarantee
an ideal pregnancy. In fact, many people, including athletes, coaches
and health care providers, may not realize that what you do prior to your
pregnancy can potentially benefit your overall pregnancy experience
and your ability to continue training comfortably. So, if your plan is to
continue with some form of training and maximize your comfort level
during your pregnancy, you may want to pay attention to our 3 "pre-
conception priorities":

- Pelvic stability
- Core strength
- Flexibility

You will be one step ahead of the game if you incorporate these elements into your regular exercise routine, sooner rather than later. You may be surprised at the impact several small changes can have on minimizing pregnancy-related discomforts while making you a stronger athlete on your journey to motherhood. In the meantime, such changes may end up making you a stronger athlete.

Pelvic Stability
The pelvis is the largest bony part of the skeleton and contains 3 joints: the pubic symphysis and 2 sacroiliac joints (Figure 2.0). A strong network of muscles and ligaments surround these joints, giving them tremendous strength. Pelvic stability refers to the ability of the torso (also known as the trunk), the hip, the pelvis and the surrounding muscles to keep the spine and pelvis in optimal alignment during your day-to-day activities and when you exercise.

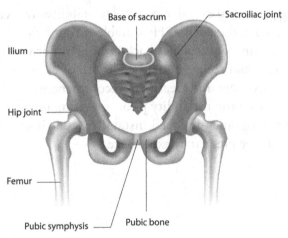

Figure 2.0 Pelvic Joints

It is not uncommon for many athletes to have some degree of pelvic instability given the repetitive and weight-bearing properties of certain sports and/or muscle imbalance or weakness in areas such as the core or lower limb. If this instability or imbalance goes untreated, pain and/or injuries will often prevail. Some of the more common signs and/or symptoms of pelvic instability include:

- Pain in the buttock region, typically on one side

- Radiating pain in the front of the pelvis, hips and/or down the back of the thigh
- Weakness with less tolerance for weight bearing on one or both legs

During your pregnancy, the risk of pelvic instability increases as a result of the numerous physical and hormonal changes to your body. One such change is the increased production of the hormone relaxin, which is responsible for relaxing the joints in preparation for childbirth. As a result, your joints became less stable and more prone to injury. This may lead to pain and discomfort, interfering with your day-to-day activities and exercise. Hale and Mile (1996) cautioned that pelvic instability might be more problematic if you continue to train at a higher level during your pregnancy. To prevent injuries, they recommend reducing your activity level, rather than trying to compensate for any instability.

How do you know if you are experiencing any pelvic instability? A good starting point is to examine your pelvic stability yourself using the method described in the sidebar "How Stable Is Your Pelvis?" Should you experience any symptoms such as back or hip pain or weakness in the leg(s), we recommend seeing a qualified health or exercise professional for a proper assessment and treatment recommendations. Taking the time *now* to correct any instability prior to getting pregnant may help minimize any pregnancy-induced instability, contributing to a more enjoyable and active pregnancy experience.

How Stable is Your Pelvis?

Here are a few simple tests to check for pelvic instability, while standing in front of a mirror.

1. Stand on one leg while trying to keep your hip bones level. If your hips are uneven when standing on one foot, you may be experiencing some sort of issue that could ultimately affect your pelvic stability. Repeat on other side. Now proceed to the next test.
2. Stand on one leg, then bend slightly at the hip and knee so that you are performing a quarter squat (i.e. doing a curtsey in front of the queen). Look to see if your knee tracks over your second toe. If the knee does not track properly over the second toe and falls inwards, it can also suggest some sort of issue that may ultimately affect your pelvic stability. Repeat on the other side. Now proceed to the next test.
3. Stand with your feet slightly wider than hip width apart. Cross your hands over your chest and perform a squat (i.e. trying to sit on an imaginary chair). As you squat into a sitting position, your back should remain neutral (meaning the curve in your back should be maintained while doing the squat) and your hips should not shift to one side. Any bending forward at the hips or shifting in the hips could also indicate some sort of issue that could ultimately affect your pelvic stability.

Any suspected pelvic instability should be followed up with a qualified health care provider, such as a sport medicine physician, physiotherapist or chiropractor.

Core Strength

Core strength tends to be the latest buzzword in training these days, especially since many studies have shown that core strength helps not only to improve athletic performance, but also day-to-day pursuits. There are two popular misunderstandings when it comes to core strength. The first misunderstanding is that many people are fooled by the appearance of a nicely toned stomach or the presence of a "six-pack" and equating it with having a strong core. However, a nicely shaped abdomen does not guarantee *functional* core strength – that is, the core strength required to support you in your sport and day-to-day activities. For instance, a runner who is fairly lean and has nicely defined abs may actually have inadequate core strength which can manifest itself in a variety of conditions, including pelvic instability, improper running style, incontinence and low back pain.

This brings us to the second common misunderstanding; when people hear the term "core strength," they tend to think of only their abdominal muscles:

- The rectus abdominis (also known as your six-pack)
- The internal/external obliques (also known as your love handles)
- The transverse abdominis (also known as your lower abs)

However, core strength involves much more than just these. In fact, it also includes the muscles from your hips to your shoulders, including your lower back, hip, buttocks and pelvic floor muscles (Figure 2.1). When engaging in most forms of activities, these muscles work together to stabilize the spine, pelvis and shoulder, creating a solid base of support.

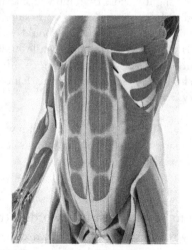

Figure 2.1 Core Muscles

Your core muscles become increasingly important during pregnancy, as they will be working even harder to accommodate the pregnancy-related changes. For instance, they will support your expanding belly while promoting proper posture and possibly minimizing any aches and pains that may occur. More importantly, your core muscles will be essential when it comes time to push during labour.

Establishing a solid core strength routine is quick and simple. Fortunately, there is an abundance of information readily available to help you do this, including books, DVDs and specialized classes at your local fitness centre. Alternatively, you can speak to a qualified exercise professional, coach or other knowledgeable health care provider for some suggestions tailored to your individual needs.

Flexibility

Flexibility, or the ease in which your joints move through a full range of motion, is another important consideration for athletes prior to getting pregnant. Some athletes may falsely assume that poor flexibility is an inevitable part of training and may not give it much attention. But not focusing on your flexibility can be problematic. In addition to feeling sore and stiff, poor flexibility can limit the way that your joints move. Consider for a moment trying to perform

> **My Story: Great Advice!**
> Tania Jones, one of Canada's fastest marathoners and mother of 2, gave me great advice: to ensure adequate core strength and balance before getting pregnant. This was the first time that I had given thought as to what I could do to better prepare my body ahead of time. I soon started working with a personal trainer and quickly discovered that my core strength and balance were not as good as I thought they were. I found the sessions so valuable that I continued working with my trainer throughout my pregnancy.
> *Jennifer Faraone, co-author, competitive duathlete and runner, mother of 2*

a squat (or similar motion to sitting in a chair) when your lower back or hip muscles are tight. Not surprisingly, you probably cannot complete the full range of motion and end up compensating (using other muscles to perform the exercise). Not only does this limit getting the most out of the activity, this compensation can increase your risk of injury.

This risk is potentially greater during your pregnancy, given that your pregnant body experiences a number of postural changes, such as the shift in the centre of your gravity and the increasing curvatures of the spine. Making your flexibility a priority prior to getting pregnant can be beneficial for a number of reasons. The first reason is that this will give you ample time to develop some form of stretching routine and improve your overall flexibility. The good news is that the routine does not have to be complicated or lengthy. In fact, your body may respond better if you target a few specific stretching exercises that you can do regularly, as opposed to attending a yoga class once a week. This could include stretching for 5-10 minutes after each workout, stretching every day while watching television or practicing yoga for 15 minutes, 3-4 times a week. Getting into a new routine now will increase the likelihood of sticking with it throughout your pregnancy.

Second, think about how great increasing your flexibility will make your body feel and move, enabling you to start your pregnancy off on the right foot. As the upcoming chapter "The Pregnant Athlete's Body" explains, your body will be going through some significant physical changes including the rounding of the shoulders, a shift in your centre of gravity and the increasing curvatures of the spine. Consider for a moment the amount of time you spend in a slouched position while sitting at a desk all day, or the number of times you bend over during the day to tie your shoes or to pick up toys off the floor. Such physical changes could place more stress on your joints and muscles, in this case your chest and mid back muscles, resulting in increased soreness and/or limited movement (Appendix 7 "Stop Breaking Your (Upper) Back, Baby" provides helpful suggestions for this particular example). Getting into the habit of stretching on a regular basis *now* and improving your flexibility may help lessen the overall impact of the pregnancy-related changes to come.

Finally, if you need more convincing about the importance of flexibility, consider your upcoming labour: a more flexible body will allow pelvis and hips to open up further, allowing you to try additional birthing positions so that your baby can pass through the birth canal with more ease.

> **My Story: My Screaming Hip Flexors**
> As an athlete, I was accustomed to having tight muscles; however I was not expecting this tightness – specifically my tight hip flexors- to interfere with my labour. Yet when it came time to pull my knees up and push, I had a very hard time holding the pose, as my hip flexors were hurting and kept cramping. It made labour even more difficult. This could have perhaps been avoided or lessened had I taken the time to stretch on a daily basis.
> *Jennifer Faraone, co-author, competitive duathlete and runner, mother of 2*

Summary

Being a strong athlete can work to your advantage but it does not guarantee that you will have a fit and/or injury-free pregnancy. Focusing on pelvis stability, strengthening your core and improving your flexibility prior to getting pregnant can certainly help. Combined, these 3 strategies may enhance your overall pregnancy experience and increase your chances of being able to train comfortably throughout all 9 months.

TRAINING FOR TWO

Chapter 3

THE PREGNANT ATHLETE'S BODY

What are the main changes my body will experience?
How will these pregnancy-related changes affect my training?
Am I okay with the amount of weight I should be gaining?

Understanding Your Changing Body

Pregnancy is one of life's most amazing miracles. It is mind-boggling to think that after an egg meets a sperm, a little person grows inside of you over the course of the next 9 months. During these magical months, your body becomes this incredible "rental unit", going through its own transformation in order to create a welcoming environment for your baby to flourish. In addition to the more obvious ways that your body transforms, such as your growing belly and the added weight, there are a number of other changes that may go unnoticed initially, including hormonal and cardiovascular changes. Such changes will likely have implications on your ability to exercise, not to mention your daily activities and may also create some mixed feelings about your new, yet temporary, body.

Understanding these changes and their implications will give you a deeper appreciation of your body's transformation. In turn, it may make it easier to listen and respond to what your body is telling you, possibly helping to minimize or prevent

> **I Knew I Was Pregnant When...**
> Over the past years of training and racing, I have come to really understand my body and how it responds to the weather, race conditions, lack of sleep, etc. So when I missed my period by one day and my boobs were extremely sore...I knew RIGHT AWAY that I was pregnant.
> *Annette Carling, triathlete and mother of 1*

discomfort and injuries. Furthermore, this knowledge may help you to embrace your changing body and provide some reassurance that, with a little time and effort, your athletic body will be back before you know it!

Your Pregnant Body's Effect on Training
The following table lists some of the more common changes that you may encounter during your pregnancy (Table 3.0). Just as no two women are alike, each pregnant athlete will have different experiences; the changes you encounter and the extent to which it affects your ability to exercise will likely differ from another expectant mom. Although the changes that come along with pregnancy may seem a bit daunting at times, the good news is that they do not necessarily mean that you need to stop exercising. You simply need to be aware of them and learn a few simple tips to help alleviate their symptoms and minimize the risk of injury.

> **Exercise Caution with Famous Expressions**
>
> Whoever came up with the expression "barefoot and pregnant" most likely was not a physiotherapist, chiropractor or other type of health care provider. According to Dr. Kevin Jardine, co-owner and rehab specialist at the sport clinic Urban Athlete, "a pregnant woman should be thinking twice about walking around barefoot during this time. Now, more than ever, she should be wearing supportive shoes as much as possible, even when she is walking around the house." Wearing proper shoes will help to counterbalance the flattening and pronation (inward collapsing) of the foot that a number of pregnant women experience. Although many women wear supportive shoes when out for a run or a long walk, they may not realize that supportive footwear is also important for all daily activities, including at home or at work.

Table 3.0: Pregnancy Changes and Potential Implications for Exercising

What You May Notice	Potential Implications For Exercising
ENERGY LEVELS	
Your body is trying to adapt to the initial changes of pregnancy, often resulting in fatigue, nausea and vomiting. These symptoms often diminish or disappear in the 2nd trimester.	• It may be difficult to find the energy to get out of bed, let alone exercise. Try a gentle form of exercise, such as walking or light spinning, rather than something more strenuous. You may feel fine once you get moving and become more energized for the remainder of the day. However, if you do not think that you could tolerate even just a few minutes, it is best to listen to your body and rest. • **Tip:** Nibbling on something light, such as crackers before and during your workout, can help with nausea. Some women have found that their nausea diminishes or disappears during their workouts.
HORMONE RELAXIN	
Your pregnant body produces more of the hormone relaxin. Its primary role is to relax the pelvic joint and ligaments in preparation for childbirth; however, it can affect all joints in the body. The elevated hormone peaks around 12 weeks, decreases in the 2nd trimester and remains stable until childbirth. The levels gradually decrease after giving birth but the effects of relaxin on your ligaments may still be evident for months afterwards.	• You may feel a bit more "loose" and unstable in any joint of the body, particularly the pelvis region. The increase of this hormone may also lead to joint pain, especially in the pelvis and low back. • **Tip:** Stretch to the point of tension or to the position that you feel the stretch, rather than overstretching and potentially hurting yourself.

HEART RATE

Due to the pregnancy-related shifts in your body, your heart rate will change throughout each trimester.

In the early stage, your resting heart rate will increase about 10-20 beats/minute, making your exercising heart rate also higher.

As your pregnancy progresses, your resting heart rate will still be elevated. However, your body adapts and your exercising heart rate more closely reflects your pre-pregnancy level.

Later in your pregnancy, your pregnant body becomes more efficient at getting blood to your working muscles, making it harder to elevate your exercising heart rate.

- You may feel a shortness of breath or a rapid heart rate. In the beginning, you might find it quite hard to keep your heart rate down, even during an easy cardiovascular workout. This should improve to some extent as your pregnancy progresses and your body becomes used to your pregnant state.
- **Tip:** Your heart rate becomes a less reliable method for monitoring your exercising intensity. This reinforces the importance of also using the Talk Test and Borg's Rating Scale of Perceived Exertion. Refer to the chapter "How Hard, How Often and How Long?" for details.

CARDIOVASCULAR SYSTEM

During pregnancy, your cardiovascular system must work harder to circulate blood and oxygen throughout your body. This is the reason for the heart rate changes mentioned above.

- You may feel lightheaded or a shortness of breath more easily.
- **Tip:** Your body needs a chance to "change gears" and adapt to the new cardiovascular demands. A longer warm up and cool down may be required.

RESPIRATORY SYSTEM

Your growing uterus pushes on your diaphragm and expands your ribcage. Breathing becomes slightly more difficult, especially when trying to take in a deep breath.

- You may feel out of breath quicker when exercising, especially in the later part of your pregnancy.
- **Tip:** You may have to adjust your workouts to accommodate your breathing.

LOWER BACK

Lower back pain during pregnancy is quite common. A number of reasons may contribute to this back pain, including maternal weight gain, joint laxity, postural changes and weak abdominal muscles.

- Experiencing pain in your lower back can significantly limit your ability to exercise, as well as interfere with daily activities.
- **Tip:** A strong core and good posture can help to alleviate the pain. You may find relief with a lower lumbar support belt (also known as the belly bra).

CENTRE OF GRAVITY	
Your centre of gravity shifts as your belly grows and can affect your sense of balance. Your "pregnancy waddle" is a way to compensate for this decreased sense of balance.	• You have an increased risk of falling or becoming off balance while doing certain types of sports and exercises including cycling, skiing, BOSU balance and lunges. • **Tip:** Extra caution is important when working out. You may want to consider modifying or replacing certain activities.
BREASTS	
Your breasts may grow in size and become tender, while your nipples and areola may darken. Such changes are due to hormonal shifts in preparation for breastfeeding.	• Exercising, especially high impact activities may be less comfortable. • **Tip:** A well-fitting and supportive bra is essential and you may find it helpful to seek out brands that make sport maternity bras. Some women also find it helpful to wear 2 bras at once.
FEET	
Your feet may seem bigger as your pregnancy progresses. This is usually a result of your weight gain, an increase in fluid (swelling) and/or soft tissue (fat). The arch in your foot may decrease (a condition referred to as "flat footedness") and your foot may be more prone to rolling inwards (referred to as "pronation") as you walk. Over time, this may cause aches and pains in the lower body and/or back.	• You may notice tenderness and pain in your feet during daily activities and when exercising and/or the need for more support. This can lead to discomfort or injuries. • **Tip:** You may want to consider wearing shoes that offer more support, possibly even orthotics.

POSTURE	
A series of postural changes usually start around week 14, with more pronounced changes later on. These changes include: • The lumbar or low back increases its lordosis (inward curve), likely due to the increased weight it must support. • The thoracic spine or upper back increases its kyphosis (outward curve) as your shoulders tend to roll forward due to the increased breast size. • The cervical spine or neck also increases its lordotic curve (by jutting the head forward) in response to the lumbar and thoracic changes.	• Although such changes are avoidable, they may affect the way that you exercise and result in more aches and pains. • **Tip:** Simply being aware of these postural changes can be helpful. Strengthening and stretching the appropriate muscles and maintaining good posture can help to relieve some of the discomfort.
ABDOMINAL MUSCLES	
Your abdominal muscles stretch as your belly expands to accommodate your growing baby. As a result, your abdominal muscles may weaken during this time and could potentially lead to diastasis recti (the separation of your abdominal muscles).	• Weak abdominal muscles may cause low back pain or other injuries. • **Tip:** It is important to continue with modified versions of abdominal strengthening activities, as long as you do not experience diastasis recti. Refer to the chapter "Your Strong And Powerful Core" for more information.
BLOOD FLOW	
When lying on your back, the weight of your enlarged uterus can press on a major vein (the inferior vena cava) and decrease blood flow to a major artery (abdominal aorta).	• You may feel lightheaded when lying on your back, especially after the 4th month. • **Tip:** Exercises normally performed on your back can be done in an upright or side-lying position. Placing a wedge under your right side or lying on an exercise ball while exercising are good options.

BODY TEMPERATURE

Your body temperature increases as a result of your pregnancy-related changes, including fluctuating hormones. Despite this increase, your temperature is still lower than that of your baby's. This difference in temperature allows your body to play a protective role for your baby; your body is able to take away any additional heat that your baby may experience at certain times, such as when fighting an infection. However, there is concern that this protective role may be diminished when your own temperature becomes too high such as during hard exercise. It is the reason sitting in a sauna or whirlpool for a prolonged period of time is contraindicated during pregnancy.	• You may feel warmer at a faster rate when exercising. This could make you feel uncomfortable and possibly nauseous. • **Tip:** Exercise in well-ventilated areas or outdoors when the temperature is favourable. It is suggested to avoid letting your body temperature exceed 38.9°C or 102°F when exercising.

The table above is not intended to detail every change your body may possibly experience and their implications on your ability to exercise. The key here is to listen to your body and to take it one day at a time.

Embracing the Weight Gain

Weight gain is another inevitable, yet crucial, component of pregnancy. Nevertheless, it can be one of the more difficult changes to accept. On one hand, you may be excited about not having to be as disciplined with your weight (and possibly your eating habits) for 9 months. On the other hand, you may experience some reservation,

Why Do I Have More Vaginal Discharge?

Have you noticed an increase in vaginal discharge now that you are pregnant? If so, relax. It is most likely leucorrhea –the same odourless or mild-smelling milky discharge that many women experience prior to pregnancy. Pregnancy just happens to produce a lot more of it, as a result of hormonal changes and greater blood flow to the vaginal area. There is not much you can do about it, other than wearing a panty liner to absorb the flow. However, if the discharge has a different colour or causes a lot of discomfort, soreness, itching or pain, contact your health care provider to rule out an infection. If you experience a large amount of thin, clear discharge, you will want to have this examined by your primary health care provider to rule out any leakage of your amniotic fluid or mucus plug.

fear or anxiety toward gaining weight, especially if you were "lean and trim" prior to getting pregnant. Your 1st trimester can be particularly challenging, as this is when you may feel more bloated but yet do not have the nicely defined "pregnancy bump". Furthermore, you may also be concerned about the impact that weight gain may have on your fitness or performance levels or have fears about losing the weight postpartum.

Rest assured, weight gain is not only a normal and healthy aspect of pregnancy, but it is also a *necessity*. It serves a very specific purpose: to supply the required energy for your baby to grow! Your growing baby needs energy 24/7 from the time of conception to the time of delivery. This energy comes directly from your weight gain. Although your baby's energy requirement is very minimal in the early stages of pregnancy, this period is when weight gain is crucial as your body is creating a "reserve of fat stores". Your baby will draw from these fat stores as their energy requirements increase throughout pregnancy.

Failure to gain an appropriate amount of weight can be problematic in more ways than one. In fact, the American Pregnancy Association cautions that an inadequate weight gain could lead to serious consequences for your baby, including malnourishment, low birth weight or premature delivery. So, as hard as it may be, embrace the fact that this is one of the few times in life when extra weight is considered a necessity! Fiona Whitby, a professional Ironman triathlete and mother of 1, found her weight gain during pregnancy to be fascinating. "It was incredible to watch my body transform and gain weight; I simply accepted that "it was what it was" and that my body knew what it needed to do in order to grow a baby."

> **It Takes Energy to Create a Healthy Baby!**
>
> Many women understand the basic need of increasing their calorie intake during pregnancy. But did you know that it takes on average 54,000-75,000 calories to make a baby? That's a lot of energy! Tara Postnikoff, Holistic Nutritionist and Personal Trainer, explains that your pregnant body needs the additional nutrients in order to support the physiological changes that are happening to both you and your baby. It is for this reason that the average pregnant woman needs to consume an additional 200-350 calories per day (above the typical daily calorie intake) and even more if she is active. Refer to the chapter "Eating for the Pregnant Athlete" for additional information about the amount of calories and nutrients required.

How much weight should you gain? As a general rule of thumb, Health Canada recommends the amount gained should be based on your pre-pregnancy weight or more specifically, your Body Mass Index (BMI) (Table 3.1). In general, women who are leaner may require more weight gain than women who are overweight prior to pregnancy; a woman carrying extra weight before pregnancy already has much of the energy stores required for pregnancy.

Table 3.1: Recommended Weight Gain in Pregnancy

Pre-Pregnancy BMI Category	Recommended Range of Total Weight Gain
<18.5	28-40 lbs.
18.5-24.9	25-35 lbs.
25.0-29.9	15-25 lbs.
≥30	11-20 lbs.

Source: ©All rights reserved. Canadian Guidelines for Body Weight Classification in Adults. Health Canada, 2003. Adapted and reproduced with permission from the Minister of Health, 2003.

Source: ©All rights reserved. Prenatal Nutrition Guidelines for Health Professionals: Gestational Weight Gain. Health Canada, 2010. Reproduced with permission from the Minister of Health, 2014.

Strategies that Can Help

Are there ideas or suggestions that can help you deal with any anxiety you may have toward gaining weight? Definitely! As a starting point, it is important to be honest with yourself and to acknowledge your concerns about your changing body and the weight gain to come. Acknowledging such feelings will help you be more open to the suggestions listed below.

Look at the Bigger Picture

Try to put things into perspective. This added weight is for a relatively short time and serves a very important purpose: to grow a healthy baby. View this time as a little "vacation" where you let yourself relax and appreciate your changing body. Learn to love your expanding belly, knowing that it is providing a cushioning and spacious environment for your baby. Appreciate the way that your breasts are changing in preparation for motherhood and breastfeeding. Most importantly, accept all the other changes that your body is going through, knowing that your body is simply doing what it needs to do in order to create a beautiful and healthy baby.

Trust and Listen to Your Body
Your body does a great job telling you what it needs and this applies to nutrition. Your increasing appetite and/or feeling of hunger may be your body's way of telling you that you need to consume additional calories and fluids. Keep in mind that the exact amount of additional calories required varies from woman to woman and depends on your level of exercise. It is therefore important that you listen to these cues and respond to them accordingly. This shall be discussed more in the chapter "Fuelling Your Pregnant Body".

It's Just a Number
Keep in mind that the numbers provided in Table 3.1 are guidelines and may not apply to everyone. Trish Del Sorbo, former owner and director of Baby & Me Fitness, suggests trusting that your body knows what it needs to do during pregnancy. In other words, if your weight gain does not match the recommended amount (either more or less) but you are eating a balanced diet and you are active - relax! Your body might simply be responding to what it needs to create the proper environment for your baby. "I found it hard mentally to accept the weight gain, especially as my weight approached that of my husband's," explains Seana Zelazo, Olympic trial marathoner and mother of 1. "I just told myself that since I was being so healthy, that this must be exactly what my son needs."

It is impossible to accurately predict the amount of weight you will gain during your pregnancy, as each woman is unique and various factors may affect the total amount gained. Examples of such factors include your pre-pregnancy weight, medical conditions, hormonal changes and the number of children you are carrying. Furthermore, exercising regularly and eating appropriately does not guarantee that your weight gain will be within the recommended guidelines (although it certainly helps!). To further illustrate the variance of weight gain, take a look at the following list describing the amount of weight gained by various high performance athletes (Table 3.2).

Table 3.2: Variations in Amount Gained During Pregnancy

Athlete	Pre-Pregnancy Weight (lbs.)	Weight Gained (lbs.)
Tara Professional Ironman Triathlete	130	35
Jessica Olympic Heptathlete	140	40
Jennifer Elite runner (pregnant with twins)	115	70
Christine Elite runner	115	60
Morgan Competitive swimmer	160	22
Karen Olympic Trampolinist	129	35
Seana Olympic Trial Marathoner	136	28

That being said, if you are finding yourself pre-occupied with your weight gain, we suggest throwing away the scale and concentrating on how you are feeling throughout your pregnancy. Fiona Whitby, referred to earlier, bought some of her favourite clothes in larger sizes, enabling her to feel better about herself and worry less about the weight gain. Rest assured that your primary health care provider will be monitoring your weight gain (or lack of) on a regular basis. If you need to lose or gain weight, they will be the first to let you know! Use your energy to ensure that you are eating a well-balanced diet and remain active. Krista DuChene, one of Canada's top marathoners, a registered dietitian and mother of 3, believes it is important to be aware of your weight but to not let it consume you.

Believe in Yourself
Remember that the changes you are experiencing are temporary. Trust that you will have the discipline once the baby is born to get yourself back into a routine with exercise and proper nutrition. Once this happens, you will soon see positive results and your pre-pregnancy body will be back in no time. Jessica Zelinka, a Canadian Olympic

heptathlete, 100m hurdler and mother of 1, became pregnant after competing in the 2008 summer Olympics and was not bothered by the 40 lbs. she gained during her pregnancy. In fact, she felt very attractive and "womanly" throughout her pregnancy. This says a lot for a person who is known across the country for her abs of steel and her extremely lean and muscular body! Jessica feels that her positive response to her weight gain had much to do with the simple fact that she (and her coach) had full confidence in her ability to return to training and lose the weight after the baby was born.

If the above strategies are not helpful and you find yourself struggling to accept your weight gain, we strongly encourage that you speak to someone, such as your doctor, a loved one or councillor about your thoughts and fears.

Summary

Your body undergoes some amazing changes during pregnancy and creates a nurturing environment for your growing baby. Not surprisingly, such changes can have implications for your daily activities and your exercise routine. Gaining a better understanding of the changes and applying some of the suggestions outlined throughout the chapter can help manage and embrace the many transformations that come with pregnancy.

Chapter 4

EXERCISE AND PREGNANCY 101

Why is it important to continue exercising now that I am pregnant?
How much is known about the safety of exercising during pregnancy?
Are there general guidelines that I should be following?

Why Exercise During Pregnancy?
Exercise plays an important role in the lives of many people, including women. Although the nature of the sport and the intensity in which one participates may vary from person to person, the reasons we exercise may be similar: to achieve or maintain good health, to feel better about ourselves and our body, to socialize with others, to be part of a team, to challenge ourselves and/or to de-stress or unwind. Such reasons likely still apply now that you are pregnant; but in case you needed more reasons, consider the *additional* benefits brought about by exercising during this time:

- Reduces backaches, constipation, bloating and swelling.
- Helps prevent or treat gestational diabetes.
- Prevents excessive weight gain.
- Increases your energy.
- Improves your mood.
- Improves your posture.
- Promotes muscle tone, strength and endurance.

> **More Great News**
> In case you needed even more reason to exercise: Canadian researchers at the University of Montreal found that exercising as little as 20 minutes a day, 3 times a week during pregnancy was enough to enhance a newborn's brain development. What a great way to give your baby a head start.

- Assists with healthy sleep patterns.
- Improves your ability to cope with labour.

No wonder many women choose to exercise throughout their pregnancy. Maybe a more appropriate question should be "*Why are you NOT exercising during pregnancy*"?

What We Know About Exercise and Pregnancy

Compared with 30 years ago, we know a lot more about exercise and pregnancy today. Generally speaking, ***most women can exercise during their pregnancy.*** In fact, being sedentary can actually lead to a number of problems including gestational diabetes, varicose veins and preeclampsia, to name a few. Here is what we do know:

- Experts recommend that women who are experiencing a healthy, low risk pregnancy participate in some form of exercise.
- For the most part, healthy pregnant women may continue an already-established exercise routine.
- For women who are continuing their regular exercise routine during pregnancy, the exercise intensity should not exceed their pre-pregnancy levels.
- No research indicates that *moderate* exercise is harmful to a developing fetus, provided that she does not exercise to exhaustion and pays attention to any warning signs from her body.

When Exercising is Not a Good Idea
There are certain reasons or circumstances, otherwise known as "contraindications", in which pregnant women should not be exercising. These contraindications can be referred to as either "absolute" or "relative". Absolute contraindication means that under *no circumstance* should you be exercising. Relative contraindication means that you and your doctor should discuss the risks and benefits of continuing to exercise should you experience certain symptoms or conditions. More detailed information on the types of contraindications can be found in the chapter "To Train or Not To Train".

- Experts have determined specific instances or conditions when it may not be a good idea to exercise; this usually only applies to a small percentage of pregnant women. These are referred to as contraindications and shall be discussed in more detail in the chapter "To Train or Not to Train".

- No research has looked at running exclusively and deemed it as an inappropriate form of exercise during a healthy pregnancy.

This increase in knowledge bodes well for pregnant women who want to continue exercising and/or training. However, this list just skims the surface of what is actually known. But how do you (and others including health care providers and exercise professionals) access such information? More importantly, how do you translate the research findings into meaningful information to help determine an appropriate amount and type of exercise while pregnant? This is where the guidelines on exercise and pregnancy come into play.

Key Concerns with Exercising
The guidelines exist to protect you and your baby. However part of making an informed decision about whether or not to exercise during your pregnancy includes understanding the potential risks.

Potential risks for the baby:

- **Hyperthermia** - higher than normal body temperature, which in extreme cases can lead to birth defects.
- **Sports Injuries** - trauma to the placenta and/or to the baby due to an extreme blow to, or fall on, the abdomen.
- **Birth Outcome** - includes gestational age and weight at birth.

Potential risks for you:

- **Dehydration** - can make you feel unwell and lead to a fever.
- **Hyperthermia** - can also increase your baby's core temperature.
- **Hypoglycemia** - your blood sugar levels fall far below normal, limiting the nutrients delivered to your working muscles and your baby.
- **Injury** - due to the effects of the hormone relaxin on your joints.

Our intent for listing these concerns is not to scare you away from exercising; rather, our goal is to educate you so that you can make informed decisions when choosing your workouts. These concerns, and how to monitor and prevent them, are described in the chapters "The

Pregnant Athlete's Body", "How Hard, How Often and How Long?" and "Monitoring the Health of You and Your Baby".

A Review of the Guidelines

If you were to do an internet search about exercise guidelines during pregnancy, there is a good chance that you would find a number of different sources offering their ideas on what you should and should not be doing. Furthermore, it may be hard to distinguish which ones are based on current research findings and come from reliable and trusted sources versus which ones do not. Making sense of all this information can be confusing! To address these challenges and simplify things for you, we have chosen to focus on the following 2 reputable guidelines:

- The Canadian guidelines developed and published jointly by the Society of Obstetricians and Gynaecologists of Canada (SOGC) and the Canadian Society for Exercise Physiology (CSEP)
- The American guidelines developed and published by the American College (now Congress) of Obstetrics and Gynecology (ACOG)

We have chosen to highlight both of these guidelines for several reasons: they were developed by leaders within their organizations, they are practical and useful to the reader, they are local in that they represent the North American population and they are based on extensive research and will continue to be updated as new research emerges. It is worth noting that many of the other guidelines that you may come across are more often than not are derived from 1 of these 2 sources.

Comparisons from Around the World

In 2013, Evenson and colleagues reviewed 11 guidelines and expert consensus from 9 countries to determine best practices and hopefully develop global recommendations for physical activity during pregnancy. The countries were: Australia, Canada, Denmark, France, Japan, Norway, Span, the United Kingdom and the United States. Although some differences were found, the authors found many positive commonalities including:

• Most guidelines support moderate-intensity physical activity during pregnancy.
• Most guidelines suggest women seek advice from their health care practitioner before starting or continuing an exercise program.
• All ruled out sports that could involve falls, trauma or collisions during pregnancy.
• Most guidelines included specific types, frequency and duration of physical activity or exercise during pregnancy.

The underlining message from this study is that women should workout during pregnancy *and* that a higher priority should be placed on promoting physical activity during pregnancy, including education and addressing barriers to physical activities.

The following table provides a summary of the general recommendations of each guideline (Table 4.1). In general, both guidelines advocate that all healthy women, in the absence of medical or obstetric complications, participate in regular exercise during pregnancy. Furthermore, both guidelines encourage a wide range of aerobic activities with some sport-specific restrictions and advise that pregnancy is not the time for achieving peak fitness or engaging in strenuous competition.

Although the underlying message is similar, you will notice a few differences among the guidelines. The Canadian guidelines seem to be more detailed and prescriptive in nature. For example, they encourage a combination of the modified age-corrected heart rate training zone, the Rating of Perceived Exertion (RPE) and the talk test when determining appropriate workout intensity. The American guidelines, on the other hand, simply suggest working out at a "moderate" level. The American guidelines are also a bit more lenient with respect to how often you should exercise. For example, the American guidelines promote regular physical activity on most, if not all days of the week, whereas the Canadian guidelines limit the frequency to 3-4 days per week. Such differences among the guidelines do not mean that one is more valid than the other; rather, it simply means that each country interpreted the data to the best of their ability and established their recommendations accordingly. So go ahead, take a few minutes to review both sets of guidelines and see how well they answered your questions.

Table 4.1: Summary of Exercise Guidelines During Pregnancy

SOGC/CSEP 2003	ACOG 2002 (reaffirmed in 2009)
GENERAL GUIDELINES	
• Women without contraindications are encouraged to participate in aerobic and strength-conditioning exercises. • The goal should be to maintain a good fitness level throughout pregnancy without trying to reach peak fitness or train for an athletic competition. • Exercises normally performed while lying on the back should be altered after the 4th month. • Activities that minimize the loss of balance and fetal trauma are recommended. • Women should be informed that exercise does not result in harmful effects on the mother and baby.	• 30 minutes or more of moderate exercise per day on most, if not all days of the week is recommended for women without contraindications. • Recreational and competitive athletes with healthy pregnancies can remain active and should modify their usual exercise routines as required. • A wide range of recreational activities appears safe; however, each sport should be reviewed for its potential risk. • Exercises performed while lying on the back and motionless standing should be minimized. • Previously inactive women and those with contraindications should be evaluated before recommendations for physical activity during pregnancy are made. • A physically active woman with a history of, or risk for, preterm delivery or intrauterine growth restriction should reduce her activity in the 2nd and 3rd trimesters.

INTENSITY	
• Modified age-corrected heart rate target zones • Talk Test • Borg's Rating of Perceived Exertion	• Moderate intensity is safe
FREQUENCY	
• 3-4 times per week	• Most, if not all days of the week
DURATION PER SESSION	
• 15 (for previously sedentary women) to 30 minutes plus warm up and cool down	• 30 minutes or more plus warm up and cool down
PREFERRED ACTIVITIES	
• Brisk walking, stationary cycling, cross-country skiing, swimming or aquafit causes less stress on the body and less bouncing than running or jogging	• Walking, swimming, cycling, aerobics • Running, certain racquet sports, and strength training for women with previous experience to the sport
EXERCISES TO AVOID OR USE CAUTION	
• Scuba diving • Lying on the back after the 4th month • Horseback riding, downhill skiing, ice hockey, gymnastics, or cycling • Hiking above 8250 ft • Abdominal strengthening exercises if diastasis recti and abdominal muscle weakness are present • Yoga and Pilates have not been well researched	• Scuba diving • Activities with high potential for contact, such as ice hockey, soccer, and basketball • High risk of falling or for abdominal trauma, such as downhill skiing and vigorous racquet sports, gymnastics, water skiing, and horseback riding • Altitudes higher than 6,000 ft

WARNING SIGNS TO STOP EXERCISING	
• Vaginal bleeding • Dyspnea prior to exertion • Dizziness • Headache • Chest pain • Muscle weakness • Calf pain or swelling • Preterm labour • Decreased fetal movement • Amniotic fluid leakage	• Vaginal bleeding • Dyspnea prior to exertion • Dizziness • Headache • Chest pain • Muscle weakness • Calf pain or swelling • Preterm labour • Decreased fetal movement • Amniotic fluid leakage
ADDITIONAL CONCERNS FOR ELITE ATHLETES	
• Competition or racing is not encouraged • Additional monitoring by an experienced health care provider is recommended for elite pregnant athletes who continue to train	• Additional monitoring by an experienced health care provider is recommended for elite pregnant athletes who continue to train
OTHER	
• Recommends the *PARmed-X for Pregnancy* to assist with the initial screening and ongoing monitoring of the exercise program	

Digesting the Information

Whew! That's a lot of information to absorb, right? Nevertheless, we hope that this information has answered many of your questions, increased your knowledge and provided you with some added reassurance about what you may or may not want to do when exercising during pregnancy. Perhaps you found that one guideline appealed to you more than the other. Or perhaps you prefer to utilize information from both guidelines (or others for that matter). If this has helped, do not stop here! We encourage you to share this information with your doctor, loved ones and coaches to ensure that they are also informed of the guidelines.

Spreading the Word

Although more is known about the safety of exercising during pregnancy, we should be cautious when assuming that health care providers, let alone the population at large, are up to speed on the latest guidelines and other pertinent information. For instance, many people still question whether it is safe to run during pregnancy (the answer is "yes", in most cases) and whether your heartbeat can exceed 140 beats per minute while exercising (once again, the answer is "yes"). A study conducted in 2010 by the American College of Sports Medicine (ACSM) found that virtually all health care providers who responded to a recent survey thought that exercise is good medicine for expecting mothers. However, 60% of physicians and 86% of doctors of osteopathy were not familiar with current pregnancy exercise guidelines. One possible explanation is that new information is constantly emerging, making it difficult for health care providers to be well versed on the most current literature.

Alternatively, you may have found that the guidelines did not meet your needs entirely, nor did they answer all of your questions. Keep in mind that the guidelines are written with the general population in mind and therefore, tend to be a bit more conservative in nature. Perhaps the stated guidelines may have raised more questions such as *"Why do the Canadian guidelines recommend using targeted heart rate training zones whereas the American guidelines do not?" "Why would the American guidelines recommend exercising most days of the week when the Canadian guidelines limit the frequency to 4 days a week?" "What happens if I exercise beyond such parameters?"* Before getting too caught up in these differences, reassure yourself with the following: both sets of guidelines are correct and you cannot go wrong by following either one. Although they may differ here and there, it is important to realize that there are more similarities than differences and that they share one very important message: get moving!!!

That being said, if you still have unanswered questions and want to dig a bit further, you will likely find the information you are looking for in future chapters. As you may have realized by now, not everything is black and white (in fact there are many shades of grey!) when it comes to exercise during pregnancy. Furthermore, there may be times when you will want to go beyond the traditional guidelines. Although it is not our job to tell you what to do in such cases, our goal is to provide you with enough information about the various shades of grey and their potential risks, so that you can make informed and educated decisions for yourself.

> **Working Out with Twins**
>
> Just because there are 2 buns in the oven does not mean you have a "no exercise" pass. In fact, if you are having a healthy pregnancy and are not experiencing any contraindications, it is safe to exercise within the recommended guidelines. Keep in mind, it is important to realize that being pregnant with twins is considered a high risk pregnancy and you have a higher possibility for developing certain conditions, including preeclampsia (pregnancy-induced hypertension), placental abruption (placenta separates from the uterine wall) and premature labour. Some sources, including the 2003 Joint SOGC/ CSEP Clinical Practice Guideline, lists "twin pregnancy after 28th week" as a relative contraindication—meaning that you should discuss with your doctor whether to continue with your exercising routine. Although research on twin pregnancy and exercise is limited, it is safe to assume that your comfort and energy levels will likely force you to slow down around this time.

Summary

Exercise during pregnancy is a complicated topic that brings about different opinions, concerns and recommendations. Fortunately, many of these concerns have been addressed and guidelines established, giving women and health care providers some much needed direction. As a result, we are seeing a greater number of pregnant women engaging in some form of physical activity. Hopefully, you feel better informed and that many of your questions regarding the type, duration, intensity, frequency and overall safety of exercising have been answered. Remember, do not stop here - we encourage you to keep reading (and moving), as there is still plenty more to discuss!

Chapter 5

TO TRAIN OR NOT TO TRAIN?

Do I want to continue with some level of training now that I am pregnant?
Which factors should I consider when making my decision?
What are the warning signs or indications that I should stop training?

Helping You Make Your Decision
Engaging in some form of exercise during pregnancy is important
for many women. This is not surprising, given the associated benefits
outlined in the chapter "Exercise and Pregnancy 101". If you are reading
this book, however, there is a good chance that your definition of "some
form" of exercise may differ from others. In fact, you may be hoping to
continue with part of your training routine in the hope of minimizing
your fitness loss and returning to your sport quickly after giving birth.

Or are you? Perhaps you are beginning to wonder if this might be
a good time to take a break from your training. This could stem from
a general fatigue following months or years of hard training, fear of
not knowing how your body will react to exercise during pregnancy
or possibly, your pregnancy-related changes are causing havoc on your
body. Furthermore, there may be medical conditions that limit your
ability to exercise during pregnancy. The bottom line is that you may
have mixed feelings or uncertainty about whether to continue training
during this time.

As you can see, such a decision is not always straightforward.
Therefore, you may find it both informative and reassuring to discuss
your training intentions with your doctor, loved ones, coach and other
health/exercise professionals. Receiving feedback from a variety of

sources that have your (and your baby's) best interest at heart may prove to be very beneficial.

Your Doctor

It is important that you discuss with your doctor, obstetrician or midwife your intentions to continue training throughout your pregnancy. This discussion should include the amount and the type of exercise you are hoping to pursue, as well as your training history over the past 12 months. This is also a good time for your primary health care provider to review your training program and to discuss potential risk factors. There are a number of conditions for which it is not appropriate to continue your fitness routine. These are classified as absolute and relative contraindications to exercise and will be discussed shortly. Not sharing information regarding your fitness routine could potentially put you and your baby at risk.

Your Loved Ones

Discussing your goals and plans with your partner, family and friends who know you intimately is also valuable. They may be able to act as a sounding board and help maintain a healthy balance between your desire to train and the activities in which you engage. Part of this discussion includes taking the time to listen to any concerns or questions that they may have and determine whether their concerns are valid and based on factual information. As necessary, you might find it helpful to provide your loved ones with some additional information, even giving them this book, as a way to help address their concerns. Not having their full support may leave you with feelings of guilt and possibly even questioning your decision to continue training.

Your Coach and Health/Exercise Professionals

Although you may be waiting to share the news about your pregnancy with others, it is important that you discuss your intentions regarding training with your coach and any other health/exercise professionals right away. If they have little experience or knowledge with respect to training and pregnancy, it is highly recommended that you also work with someone that understands the pregnant athlete. Together you can work on establishing training goals that are meaningful, realistic and safe for you and your baby.

A great way to facilitate this open communication is to have your coach (or health/exercise professional) describe in detail your proposed training plan in the *PARmed-X for Pregnancy (Physical Activity Readiness Medical Examination)* as outlined in Appendix 1. Launched by the Canadian Society for Exercise Physiology (CSEP) and designed by medical doctors and researchers, this tool was developed to screen women interested in participating in physical activity during pregnancy. This simple and easy to use form also provides helpful information and guidelines regarding exercising during your pregnancy. Once you and your coach have completed the first part of the form, you can then review it with your doctor to discuss whether there are contraindications to exercising and if there are any concerns with your proposed training plan. Following the approval from your doctor, you can then bring the signed form to your coach. Not only will you, your coach and your doctor have a common understanding of your intended training plan, but it can also offer everyone reassurance that the plan is based on reasonable and knowledgeable input.

Self-Reflection
Up until now, the primary assumption has been that you *want* to continue with some form of training during pregnancy. But this may not be the case, and it does not mean that you are less of an athlete if you decide not to train during this time. Although you might have given it a lot of thought *before* getting pregnant and had every intention to maintain some level of training during your pregnancy, there is the possibility that you may now change your mind. As many women will agree, it is amazing how quickly your perspective on life can change the moment you become pregnant.

However, any intentions to reduce or discontinue your training may be overshadowed by thoughts that "I *should* be exercising". Such thoughts may stem from an internal source (e.g. your desire to preserve as much fitness as possible) or from an external source (e.g. feeling pressured from sponsors). To help understand your level and source of motivation, you may find it helpful to reflect on the following questions and to discuss them with your loved ones, coach and doctor:

- *Do I have any concerns about my training during my pregnancy?*
- *Do I want to continue training or would I rather be active if/when I feel like it?*

- *What are my reasons for wanting to train during this time?*
- *Do I feel pressured to continue training?*
- *Will I feel relieved or guilty if I decide to stop training?*

Although additional strategies and suggestions for coping with the emotional side of cutting back on your training will be discussed in the chapter "Pacing Your Mind", the immediate take-away message is this: now more than ever it is important to get past this idea that "I *should* be exercising" and to listen instead to your body, mind and heart.

> **Being Honest with Yourself and Others**
>
> Some athletes, especially those who have demonstrated a very high level of commitment to their sport, may welcome pregnancy as the opportunity to take a break from their training. If that's the case for you – congratulations for realizing this and making this decision for yourself! But equally important is that you share this decision with others.
>
> Andrea Page, founder of Andrea Page's Original Fitmom, recalls working with a pregnant Olympic athlete who suddenly stopped exercise altogether, claiming that her coach had instructed her to do so. Knowing that the athlete did not have any contraindications to exercise, Page tried explaining to her that it was safe, not to mention beneficial, for her to continue with some form of exercise. Page suspected that the break in exercise was more likely due to the athlete's level of motivation, that she was probably feeling burned out after years of strenuous training. Perhaps this athlete was looking for permission to stop training, without feeling guilty but was afraid to admit it.
>
> Such feelings are understandable but it is unfortunate that the athlete did not feel comfortable verbalizing this or perhaps could not even admit it to herself. Not only did this limit Page's working relationship with her, more importantly, she likely did not experience all the benefits of exercising during pregnancy.

When Exercising is Not a Good Idea

Despite everything that we have just discussed, there is one consideration that trumps your desire to continue training: the presence of any medical conditions that puts the health of you and your baby at risk. These medical conditions are classified as either absolute or relative contraindications. "Absolute" contradictions mean that you should not exercise if you experience any of the conditions listed. "Relative" contraindications mean that you and your doctor should discuss the risks and benefits of continuing to exercise, should you experience certain symptoms or conditions (Table 5.0).

Table 5.0: Absolute and Relative Contraindications to Exercise

Joint SOGC/CSEP Guidelines	
Absolute Contraindications	**Relative Contraindications**
• Ruptured membranes, premature labour • Persistent 2nd or 3rd trimester bleeding/placenta previa • Pregnancy-induced hypertension or preeclampsia • Incompetent cervix • Evidence of intrauterine growth restriction • High order of pregnancy (e.g. triplets) • Uncontrolled Type 1 diabetes, hypertension or thyroid disease, other serious cardiovascular, respiratory or systemic disease	• History of spontaneous abortion or premature labour in previous pregnancies • Mild/moderate cardiovascular or respiratory disease (e.g. chronic hypertension, asthma) • Anemia or iron deficiency (Hb<100g/L) • Very low body fatness, eating disorder (anorexia/bulimia) • Twin pregnancy after 28th week • Other significant medical condition
ACOG Guidelines	
Absolute Contraindications	**Relative Contraindications**
• Hemodynamically significant heart disease • Restrictive lung disease • Incompetent cervix/cerclage • Multiple gestation at risk for premature labour • Persistent 2nd or 3rd trimester bleeding • Placenta previa after 26 weeks of gestation • Premature labour during the current pregnancy • Ruptured membranes • Preeclampsia/pregnancy-induced hypertension	• Severe anemia • Unevaluated maternal cardiac arrhythmia • Chronic bronchitis • Poorly controlled type 1 diabetes • Extreme morbid obesity • Extreme underweight (BMI<12) • History of extremely sedentary lifestyle • Intrauterine growth restriction in current pregnancy • Poorly controlled hypertension • Orthopedic limitations

	• Poorly controlled seizure disorder
	• Poorly controlled hyperthyroidism
	• Heavy smoker

You may notice small differences in the suggested contraindications outlined in the Canadian guidelines compared to those listed in the American guidelines. These differences further reinforce the importance of discussing your intentions to continue training with your doctor. Together, you can decide whether the benefits outweigh the risks of being physically active. In addition to these contraindications, there are other symptoms that you should be aware of while exercising. It is important that you stop exercising immediately and seek medical attention should you experience any of these symptoms (Table 5.1).

Table 5.1: Warning Signs to Stop Exercising When Pregnant

Joint SOGC/CSEP Guidelines	ACOG Guidelines
• Excessive shortness of breath	• Vaginal bleeding
• Chest pain	• Dyspnea prior to exertion (shortness of breath)
• Presyncope (lightheadedness)	• Dizziness
• Painful uterine contractions	• Headache
• Leakage of amniotic fluid	• Chest pain
• Vaginal bleeding	• Muscle weakness
	• Calf pain or swelling
	• Preterm labour
	• Decreased fetal movement
	• Amniotic fluid leakage

Although you may have been accustomed to pushing yourself through pain in past workouts, the following can never be said enough: now more than ever, it is important to listen to your body. If it does not feel right, don't do it!

Stay Active

We have just reviewed a variety of reasons why you may decide to take a pause from your training. But this does not mean that you should be throwing in the towel altogether! Assuming that you are not on bed rest and that there are no absolute contraindications to exercise, it is strongly encouraged that you make a personal commitment of doing *some form of exercise,* a minimum of 3 times a week. This may include walking at a brisk pace, trying a new activity such as yoga or working with a qualified pre-natal fitness expert over the next 9 months.

As detailed in the chapter "Exercise and Pregnancy 101", staying physically active is extremely important during your pregnancy for several reasons:

- Enables you to build your strength and endurance for labour.
- Manages an appropriate weight gain.
- Prevents or lessens certain pregnancy-related conditions.
- Prepares you for carrying your baby and all of his/her gear postpartum.

Equally importantly, it will give you peace of mind knowing you have done something good for you and your baby. If you are not already convinced, there is one more reason for staying active during your pregnancy - completely discontinuing your exercise routine will only make your postpartum comeback much more challenging and no doubt, longer!

Summary

Deciding whether to continue training and at what level throughout your pregnancy is an individual decision that differs from woman to woman. This decision should be based on what is right for you and your baby and takes into consideration your past and current medical status (including any contraindications), your reasons for wanting to continue training, as well as any concerns or doubts that you may have. Speaking with your doctor, loved ones, coach or other health/exercise professionals will help guide your decision and provide you with some support and reassurance.

Chapter 6

HOW HARD, HOW OFTEN
AND HOW LONG?

Are hard workouts off limits?
Am I putting my baby or myself at risk if I exercise daily?
Can I exercise longer than the recommended 30 minutes?

Looking Beyond the Guidelines
As discussed in the chapter "Exercise and Pregnancy 101", there are guidelines regarding the amount and type of exercise that you can safely perform during your pregnancy. Although different sources vary, they more or less recommend the following:

- Maintain an easy-to-moderate intensity.
- Exercise a minimum of 3 days a week.
- Exercise approximately 30 minutes at a time.

Although such guidelines may suffice for the beginner or recreational exerciser, we know this information may lead to more questions for the seasoned athlete. In fact, you might already be thinking:

- *I am accustomed to a higher volume and intensity of training; I am not sure that these guidelines apply to me.*
- *I run marathons and therefore, should be able to handle running longer than 30 minutes at an easy pace.*
- *I do not typically take days off, so why should I start now?*
- *I need to do more than the recommended guidelines; otherwise, I will drive myself insane.*

Comments like these speak to the gap existing between the more conservative guidelines and the typical day-to-day workouts of many athletes. This does not mean, however, that you should assume the guidelines do not apply to you and that it is safe for you, as an experienced athlete, to do your own thing or to simply replicate another pregnant athlete's training plan. This is where this chapter comes in handy, as we explore the topic of intensity, duration and frequency of exercise during pregnancy in much greater detail. Not only will we dig deeper into the guidelines but we will also discuss some of the concerns associated with exercising beyond the guidelines. In doing so, we hope to help you make informed decisions about how to train throughout your pregnancy. This is assuming, of course, that you are experiencing a healthy pregnancy and that there are no contraindications to exercise.

Resist the Urge

It is easy to become familiar with the guidelines for exercise and pregnancy and understand the rational for why they exist. But it may be harder to apply them to yourself when you hear stories about other pregnant athletes that go above and beyond them. For instance, you may know of a woman who trained hard during her 1st trimester, only to realize later that she was pregnant. Or you may have heard of a pregnant woman that ran a marathon without experiencing any complications. You cannot help but wonder whether or not you could do the same?

As hard as it may be, we encourage you to resist the urge to plan your workouts based on what you have seen or heard from other pregnant women. First of all, the number of women described in the above scenarios is quite small, and there is also a lot of hearsay when it comes to this topic. Second, and perhaps more important, you need to realize that you are likely only hearing one piece of the story. What was this woman's training history? Did she have her doctor's approval? Did she experience complications later on? Furthermore, just because it was safe for one woman does not guarantee that it will be safe for you to engage in the same type of physical activity that goes above and beyond the recommended guidelines. Are you willing to take this risk?

The Challenge

When it comes to exercising during pregnancy, most women want to know "how hard, how often and/or how long can I work out?" Therefore, we have presented the information in the following manner: intensity, frequency and duration. The challenge with this approach, however, is that many of the research studies do not look at these variables individually, limiting our ability to analyze and compare the findings.

For instance, one study may have looked at the combined effect of intensity and frequency whereas another study may have only looked at frequency. Furthermore, even when different studies focused on the same outcome - for example, birth weight, it can be difficult to compare their findings, as the intensity, frequency and duration of the exercise under investigation likely differs between studies. Such challenges are evident when examining the following studies that focused their findings on birth outcomes:

- In 1995, Bell and colleagues examined a small number of pregnant women in their 25th week and found that those who exercised vigorously for at least 30 minutes, 4 or more times per week, had babies whose mean birth weight was significantly lower (approximately ½ lb.) compared with women who did not exercise.
- In 2002, Evenson and colleagues surveyed 1,699 women and found that participation in vigorous leisure activity (at least twice a week) prior to pregnancy, during the 1st trimester and even more so, in the 2nd trimester, was associated with a reduced risk of pre-term birth.
- In 2006, Duncombe and team conducted a small study on 148 pregnant women and found no evidence that the intensity, duration and frequency of vigorous exercise were associated with significant reductions

Why Look at Birth Outcomes?

Although there are numerous outcomes that can be considered, many studies about exercise and pregnancy often focus their findings on birth outcomes - which can include birth weight or gestational age of the infant. Why is that? Put simply, birth outcomes can tell us a lot about the health of the baby.

Low birth weight, often described as a baby born with a weight that is less than the 10th percentile, has been shown to increase the risk of short and long-term complications to both the mother (e.g. preeclampsia and premature labour) and her baby (e.g. stillbirth, respiratory distress and developmental difficulties later in life). The gestational age of the infant, also known as the time between conception and birth, is the other area of focus for many studies. Not only can it affect birth weight but a short gestational age (or preterm birth) is also the leading cause of fetal and infant death in North America and Europe, as well as a major predictor of infant illness or disease.

in either birth weight or gestational age of the infant. Vigorous exercise was looked at in terms of the type of aerobic activity, the intensity (heart rate above 140 beats per minute or at least 50% of age-adjusted heart rate), time (15-30 minutes or more of continuous activity) and frequency (at least 3 times per week).

What do the above studies tell us? They illustrate that no 2 studies are the same and that it can be challenging to obtain clearly defined answers as to how hard, how often and how long a pregnant woman can exercise. It is also worthwhile to mention that all of the researchers behind the above studies acknowledged the limitations within their studies and recommended that more robust and/or larger-scale research be conducted. So, if we do not have all the answers, how do you proceed with determining an appropriate exercise or training plan if you choose to go above and beyond the guidelines?

Our first suggestion is to reflect on WHY you want to engage in an exercise regime that extends beyond the recommended guidelines. As previously discussed in the chapter "To Train or Not To Train", you might find it helpful to reflect on the following:

- Do you have a true desire to engage in more strenuous workouts, or is this intent stemming from a sense of obligation or fear?
- Do you want to work out more often than 3 times a week because exercising also serves as a daily stress reliever, or are you trying to minimize your weight gain?
- Do you want to exercise longer than 30 minutes simply because you are accustomed to longer workouts, or is it because you feel that this will help maintain your fitness as much as possible?
- Are you able to give yourself permission to scale back on your workouts?

Our second suggestion is that you take the time to become even more knowledgeable about the 3 variables (intensity, frequency and duration), including an understanding of the potential risks associated with each one. In turn, this will empower you and perhaps your doctor, coach or anyone else on your health care team to make informed decisions about the appropriate level of exercise for you.

Increasing your knowledge however, requires providing you with an abundance of information in a simple and logical manner. We have simplified the topics by dividing the rest of the chapter into categories answering the following questions:

- *How hard can I workout (intensity)?*
- *How often can I exercise (frequency)?*
- *How long can I exercise at a time (duration)?*

We have also included other practical strategies and sample workouts that we think you will appreciate and enjoy. So get comfortable and start reading!

Above All Else

Before getting too caught up in the details surrounding how hard, how often and how long to exercise, we want to focus your attention on the following piece of advice - *make a conscious effort to listen to what your body is telling you AND to respond appropriately to its cues when exercising.* This means accepting the fact that you are no longer in control of your body during this 9-month period or in the first few months postpartum. For example, although you are accustomed to challenging workouts, you may suddenly find that your lower back and tailbone become sore the moment you try to increase the intensity of a workout, or working out on consecutive days leaves your body aching constantly, or you feel lightheaded and exhausted whenever you try to exercise beyond 30 minutes. Whatever the symptoms may be, it is important to pay attention to how your body is responding and to modify your exercise as required (Table 6.0).

Although this may sound pretty straightforward (and repetitive), we know that letting your body (and not your mind) be the driver of your workouts can be challenging, especially when your dedication to the sport is so strong. "As athletes, we are accustomed to being able to control how our bodies perform and how our bodies look; pregnancy is the one time where we need to let go of this control," says Sharon Donnelly, 3-time Canadian champion, Olympic triathlete and mother of 2. "If we can do this, our pregnancy will go more smoothly."

How Hard?

Determining and maintaining a workout intensity that is effective for you and safe for your baby can be challenging; what is considered "hard" for a pregnant woman is very different than a non-pregnant woman.

For instance, the heart rate or training zone that you were previously accustomed to may no longer apply, as such values tend to change with pregnancy. Furthermore, the term "moderate" intensity that is used in many guidelines is not always well defined and its meaning can vary from person to person. Finally, different guidelines or sources will recommend different methods, if any, for monitoring your level of intensity while exercising.

Table 6.0: Know When to Stop

Regardless of the type, volume and intensity of exercise that you engage in, there are certain symptoms that you should be on the alert for *during and after exercise*. As described in the chapter "To Train or Not to Train", you should stop exercising immediately and seek medical attention if you experience any of the following:

- Excessive shortness of breath
- Shortness of breath prior to exertion
- Headache
- Dizziness or faintness
- Chest pains
- Muscle weakness
- Calf pain or swelling
- Painful uterine contractions (more than 6-8 per hour)
- Preterm labour
- Vaginal bleeding
- Any "gush" of fluid from your vagina, amniotic fluid leakage
- Decreased fetal movement

So, how do you decide what is too hard? Fortunately, there are 5 different methods that can be used to help determine how hard (or how easy) you should be exercising while pregnant. They include:

- Talk test
- Rating of perceived exertion
- Heart rate
- Training history
- Common sense

These methods are used either independently or jointly, depending on which source is being referenced. It is not uncommon to find the first 3 methods combined, such as in the 2003 Clinical Practice Guidelines on Exercise in Pregnancy and the Postpartum Period jointly set by the Society of Obstetricians and Gynaecologists of Canada (SOGC) and the Canadian Society for Exercise Physiology (CSEP). As such, they can also be found on the *PARmed-X for Pregnancy* (Appendix 1).

Talk Test

The talk test is an informal and subjective method to determine the appropriate exercise intensity and refers to the ability to carry on a conversation while exercising. If you are not able to talk during your workout or you are gasping for air, it means that you are likely exerting yourself too much and that you should be taking your activity down a notch. Several studies, including one by Persinger and colleagues (2004), confirmed that the talk test can be used as a simple way of examining exercise intensity.

Rating of Perceived Exertion

The Borg's Rating of Perceived Exertion (RPE) chart was designed as a simple tool that can be applied to most people, regardless of gender, age, health conditions or national origin (Table 6.1). Applying the tool is easy, as it only requires you to rate your effort level (how hard you think you are working out) on a scale of 6-20. Your rating is actually influenced by the way that your body responds to exercise, such as the way that your muscles and joints feel, your breathing and your heart rate. For the reasons mentioned above, the RPE is a tool often used during pregnancy.

The 2003 SOGC/CSEP Clinical Practice Guidelines put forward the recommendation that pregnant women should stay within the RPE range of 12-14 (somewhat hard) to maintain fitness. Numerous sources have since adopted this specific recommendation, including the Canadian Academy of Sport and Exercise Medicine (CASEM) and the American College of Sports Medicine (ACSM).

Table 6.1: Borg's Rating Scale of Perceived Exertion

Exertion	RPE
No exertion at all	6
Extremely light	7
	8
Very light	9
	10
Light	11
	12
Somewhat hard*	**13**
	14
Hard (heavy)	15
	16
Very hard	17
	18
Extremely hard	19
Maximal exertion	20

*A rating of 12-14 is the recommended ranged during pregnancy.
Adapted from PARmed-X for Pregnancy, © Canadian Society of Exercise Physiology, 2013

Heart Rate

For many athletes, a more common and perhaps familiar approach is using heart rate and heart rate training zones (HRTZ). Heart rate is the number of times your heart beats per minute and HRTZ are used to define appropriate exercise intensity to elicit a training effect. Once you are pregnant, however, the values of your pre-pregnancy HRTZ are no longer valid. This is the result of the cardiovascular changes occurring in your body and their effect on your heart rate. Therefore, appropriately adjusted HRTZ are required when using this monitoring method during your pregnancy. For instance, the 2003 joint SOGC/CSEP Clinical Practice Guidelines recommends a modified version of the conventional age-corrected heart rate training zones for exercising during pregnancy (Table 6.2).

Table 6.2: Modified Heart Rate Training Zones for Aerobic Exercise in Pregnancy

Maternal Age	Heart Rate Training Zone (Beats/Minute)	Heart Rate Target Zone (Beats/10 Seconds)
Less than 20	140-155	23-26
20-29	135-150	22-25
30-39	130-145	21-24
40 or greater	125-140	20-23

Source: Joint SOGC/CSEP Clinical Practice Guideline: Exercise in Pregnancy and the Postpartum Period, 2003

More recently, new HRTZ have been established following a study led by Mottola and colleagues at Western University. They determined that fit pregnant women could safely exercise at a higher intensity than the average pregnant person (Table 6.3). These results have been incorporated into the 2013 *PARmed-X for Pregnancy* and have been adopted by the American College of Sports Medicine.

Table 6.3: Revised Modified Heart Rate Training Zones for Aerobic Exercise in Pregnancy

Age	Revised Heart Rate Training Zones (beats/minute)	Category Description
Less than 20	Not looked at in their study; use values in Table 6.2	Low – Beginner athletes Active – Recreational athletes Fit – Competitive athletes
20-29	Low 129-144 Active 135-150 Fit 145-160 BMI>25kgm^2 102-124	
30-39	Low 128-144 Active 130-145 Fit 140-156 BMI>25kgm^2 101-120	BMI – Body Mass Index (see "Training for Conception" for more information)
40 or greater	Not looked at in their study; use values in Table 6.2	

Adapted from PARmed-X for Pregnancy 2013 (Mottola et al., 2006; Davenport et al., 2008).

It is important to note that the recommendation of using heart rate as a measure of intensity varies greatly among different sources. Part of this variation can be attributed to the number of factors that may influence heart rate including:

- Environmental factors such as dehydration or poor sleep.
- The nature of the sport, as some activities will raise one's heart rate quicker than others.
- The fluctuating heart rate levels that occur throughout pregnancy.

The other part of this discrepancy stems from the initial recommendation in the early 80's that advised pregnant women to keep their heart rate under 140 beats per minute when exercising. This recommendation was part of the initial guidelines set out by the American College of Obstetricians and Gynecologists (ACOG) in 1984 and was based on the idea that elevating the heart rate raises the mother's body temperature to a level that could be harmful to the fetus. ACOG has since dropped this recommendation in their more recent guidelines and now advises pregnant women to monitor their fatigue as a way to assess their level of intensity. Despite the change to this recommendation, it is surprising how many people, including health care providers, still refer to the initial, yet outdated, guidelines of 140 beats per minute.

Lastly, there is a final consideration: your familiarity with measuring your heart rate. This can be done manually by finding your pulse and placing your 2nd and 3rd fingers on either the side of your neck (at the point where your jaw meets your neck) or on the inside of your wrist (on the thumb side). Once you have found your pulse, count the number of beats for 10 seconds. Multiply this number by 6 to determine the number of beats per minute. Another common and easier way to measure heart rate is to wear a heart rate monitor.

Training History

Many experts agree that one of the most valid indicators in determining your exercise intensity at this time is based on your training regime *before* getting pregnant. This includes both the type of activities (running versus swimming) and the performance level (how much you do and how hard you train). The reason for this is simple: the more that you engage in similar pre-pregnancy activities, the less of a shock it will be to your pregnant body. Furthermore, your familiarity with how your body responded to past workouts will help you gauge how much your pregnant body can now handle. For example, a runner accustomed to running speed intervals may better

Modifying the Game

Elite squash players and teammates Stephanie Hewitt and Seanna Keating have placed in the top 10 at various world championship competitions for many years, including winning gold at the World Squash Doubles Championship in 2011. So, it was pretty convenient to continue playing with (or against) each other when they became pregnant at the same time. Their motto for playing became "pick your partners and modify the game". For instance, they adopted a "2-bounce" rule and played doubles (as opposed to singles) to decrease the risk of getting injured and to reduce the amount of running back and forth. They also selected opponents who were better suited to their current playing level and who did not feel uncomfortable playing against them. "We know that there were people who were hesitant to play against us, out of fear of causing harm," said Stephanie. "But for the most part, the people at our club were very positive and supportive."

Stephanie Hewitt & Seanna Keating, elite squash players and mothers of 3

tolerate such workouts during her pregnancy, albeit less intense, than a runner accustomed to always running at a relaxed pace. This is one of the reasons it is recommended that women who are new to exercising wait until their 2nd trimester before engaging in a new exercise program. Her body is simply not used to the physical demands of exercising and it is unknown how her newly pregnant body will react to physical activity and/or its potential effect on the developing baby.

This does not mean, however, that you should simply replicate your pre-pregnancy exercise regime; in most cases, you will likely need to scale down the intensity, as well as the volume and duration. Rather, use your pre-pregnancy exercise regime as a starting point to determine what your workouts will now look like, as opposed to simply following a generic training plan or copying what another pregnant athlete did. Starting off with a program that is similar to what you were previously accustomed to may be more safe, tailored and beneficial to you and your exercise goals.

Common Sense
Regardless of whether you choose to use any of the methods discussed up until now, we encourage you to follow these basic principles when exercising:

- Avoid exercising to the point of exhaustion.
- Take the time to listen to your body; if your body is not responding well to the particular exercise, skip the activity.
- Speak up and ask questions when you have uncertainty.
- When in doubt about a particular exercise, err on the side of caution.

Simple and to the point, these principles will no doubt help to ensure that you are exercising at an appropriate intensity.

Determining Your Intensity
We hope that these methods provided some added reassurance that, yes, you can make yourself sweat by engaging in workouts of varying intensity. In fact, we even included 3 sample cardiovascular workouts at the end of this book that you might enjoy (Appendix 2). Remember - there is no magic formula that will tell you exactly how hard you can exercise, nor is there the science to identify which women can train

harder than others without experiencing any negative effects. To recap, using any or all of the following methods can help to determine an appropriate intensity for your workouts:

- Ensure that you can perform the talk test while exercising.
- Keep your RPE between 12-14.
- Monitor your heart rate according to the prescribed heart rate training zones.
- Take into account your training history.
- Let common sense guide you in your decisions.

How I Monitored My Intensity

Jean Wilson, an accomplished runner, was feeling great during her pregnancy and was even able to run 2 half marathons during this time. Although she ran both races for enjoyment, she surprised herself with how well she performed. How did she make sure that she did not exert herself too much during the race? By forgetting about the numbers (and not wearing her heart rate monitor), and paying attention to her breathing, keeping the pace relaxed and at a conversational level, and making sure that at no point was she exerting herself.

Running a half marathon during pregnancy is not something that applies to most women. However, the take away message speaks to all pregnant athletes: listening to your body, knowing your limits and lowering or removing your performance expectations are a must!

Jean Wilson, competitive runner, mother of 1

How Often?

Even something as simple as the recommended number of days a pregnant woman should exercise can vary depending on the source you reference. Consider the following:

- ACOG recommends that women with low-risk pregnancies participate in moderate-intensity physical activity on most, if not all, days of the week.
- SOGC and CSEP recommend exercising 3-4 days per week.
- CASEM recommends exercising 3 times per week progressing to a maximum of 4-5 times per week.

Why such differences? What is concerning about exercising more often? What if you were accustomed to exercising on a daily basis? There are 2 primary reasons behind these differences and limitations. The first reason has to do with what has been demonstrated in research - that exercising 3-4 days is usually safe for the mother and her baby. One way research defines "safe" is by looking at birth outcomes, such as number of pre-term births, birth weight or APGAR scores. Differences in research findings start to emerge when the frequency of exercise increases (or decreases) beyond these guidelines.

For example, a study by Campbell and Mottola (2001) found the odds of giving birth to a lower birth weight infant were substantially increased in pregnant women who engaged in structured recreational exercise 5 or more times per week during their 3rd trimester compared to those who exercised 3-4 times per week. The authors suggest that lower birth weight infants have an increased risk of short and long-term complications such as respiratory distress and developmental difficulties later in life. On the other hand, Kardel and Kase (1998) found that well-conditioned female athletes who continued to exercise 6 times per week at high-intensity throughout pregnancy gave birth to heavier newborns compared to pregnant women who exercised at a moderate-intensity. The authors of this study stated that the health of the baby was not compromised.

Finally, Leet and Flick (2003) examined 30 studies to determine whether birth weight was dependent on the mother's fitness level prior to pregnancy and how far into her pregnancy she continued to exercise. They concluded that there were minimal differences in birth weight of babies born to mothers who exercised compared to mothers who did not. However, they concluded that babies born to mothers who continued to exercise vigorously into their 3rd trimester were likely to be 200-400g lighter (compared to babies whose mother did not exercise vigorously at this point). The authors questioned whether this amount (200-400g) is clinically significant and suggested that it does not appear to put a baby's health at risk.

> **Taking It One Day (or Trimester) at a Time**
>
> Leslie Black, an experienced marathoner, intended to continue her daily runs throughout her pregnancy. Therefore, she was surprised when her extreme nausea and fatigue prevented her from getting out the door to exercise in her 1st trimester. But as her pregnancy progressed, the nausea diminished and her energy levels increased, she purchased a treadmill and began to run every second day until it became too uncomfortable in her 7th month.
>
> *Leslie Black, competitive runner and mother of 2*

Putting the research findings aside, the second reason for the limitation of frequency is for your protection. More specifically, the recommendations help to ensure that you do not overextend yourself, become fatigued and place yourself at greater risk for injury. Although you might have been accustomed to working out on a daily basis, you have to remember that being pregnant is a workout on its own; it places more cardiovascular and physical demands on your body. So, even when you are not exercising, you are, in fact, working out! You may also find that your pregnant body is in need of more rest days, in addition to decreasing the intensity and duration of your workouts. Dr. Mottola suggests that some women may benefit from alternating the number of workouts they do per week. For instance, if you went to the gym 4 times this week, your body might appreciate exercising only 3 times the following week.

Determining Your Frequency

What is the bottom line? Will exercising beyond 3 or 4 days place the health of you or your baby at risk? Not necessarily, as there is there is limited and inconclusive evidence. Therefore, we suggest the following approach when considering how often to exercise:

- Look at the number of workouts per week that you were accustomed to prior to getting pregnant and then take it down a notch - at least initially, until you see how your body responds. For instance, if you typically worked out 5 days a week and feel relatively well during your pregnancy, consider starting with 3 or 4 days a week. Both your mind and your body may appreciate the additional rest days.
- Listen to your body. Respect any variations in your energy levels and err on the side of caution when in doubt. For example, if you only had the energy to exercise 2 times a week in your 1st trimester, try to be accepting of that amount. It is possible you could increase the frequency in your 2nd trimester as your body better adapts to the demands of pregnancy and you feel less tired.
- If you want to do some form of exercise every day, consider doing a lighter activity, such as walking. This might offer the perfect balance between your desire for daily activity, while still respecting your body's need for rest.

- Consider keeping a journal to track the number and type of workouts you engage in, your energy levels and how your body feels. Sometimes it can be easier to look back and identify a particular pattern. For instance, you may notice that your energy levels were better when you limited your workouts to 3 times per week, compared to when you exercised 5 times per week.

How Long?

Duration, or the amount of time spent exercising, is another factor where there is variation, both in terms of what is recommended and what pregnant women actually do. Part of this variation may be due to the nature of the sport (e.g. an Ironman athlete versus a basketball player), the ranges within a particular sport (e.g. a marathon runner versus a sprinter) and the duration of exercise that you were accustomed to, prior to getting pregnant (e.g. cross country skiing for 3 hours versus 40 minutes).

As highlighted in the chapter "Exercise and Pregnancy 101", there are guidelines that speak to the duration of your workout. For instance, SOGC/CSEP recommends 15-30 minutes of exercise plus a warm up and cool down, whereas ACOG recommends 30 minutes or more of exercise each day. This "30 minutes or more" leaves a lot open for interpretation! If you were accustomed to training for longer than 30 minutes, you might be wondering why the Canadian guidelines place an upper limit, and what happens if you exercise beyond this.

Surely if some women ran, skied or cycled for over an hour and did not experience any maternal or fetal complications, it must be safe, right? Not necessarily. There are some reports in the literature about pregnant women participating in endurance events such as a marathon but it is important to note such reports are not considered the best evidence when determining a true cause-and-effect relationship. Furthermore, there are only a few clinical studies that have looked at what happens when a pregnant woman exercises longer than 45 minutes. Whereas it is safe to say that we understand the implications for mother and child when a pregnant woman exercises up to 45 minutes, our understanding of what happens when she exercises beyond this threshold is limited. Finally, it is not very often that a study will examine duration by itself. More often than not, other variables such as frequency or intensity are incorporated into the research. Consider the following studies:

- Lockey et al. (1991) gathered 18 of the best exercise and pregnancy research studies available and performed a comprehensive analysis (known as a meta-analysis) of their findings. After examining all the studies together, they determined that an exercise program performed on average for 43 minutes per day, 3 times per week with a heart rate up to 144 beats per minute, does not appear to cause harm to the mother or fetus in a normal healthy pregnancy.

- A Scandinavian study by Kardel (2005) looked at the effects of medium and high intensity exercise during and after pregnancy in 41 elite athletes. Part of the training regime included a bout of aerobic endurance training in which the medium and high exercise groups were assigned 1h 30 min or 2h 30 min of cycling, fast walking or cross country skiing, twice a week at low intensity (120-140 beats per minute). The results showed that women who were well trained prior to pregnancy benefit from continued training at high levels during an uncomplicated pregnancy. The authors suggested that such training may allow a more rapid return to competitive activity and healthy life after pregnancy. Furthermore, Kardel and Kase (1998) found that participating in similar activities did not compromise the baby's growth and development.

- More recently, Mottola and colleagues (2013) determined that pregnant women were able to maintain adequate blood sugar levels for the initial 30 minutes of moderate intensity exercise; these levels then dropped significantly when the time was extended to 40 minutes. Once lowered, the blood sugar levels took a while to return to an acceptable level. A low blood sugar level may be problematic during pregnancy because fewer nutrients are being delivered to the baby. Mottola further suggested that exercise up to 40 minutes appears to be well tolerated by mother and baby, however caution is warranted.

Determining Your Duration

It is safe to say that most, if not all studies have shown that 30 minutes of exercise is an acceptable duration. But what happens beyond this time remains somewhat unclear, due to a limited number of good or strong studies on this topic. If you are considering exercising for longer, we encourage you to consider the following strategies:

- Not all workouts need to be of the same duration. Consider alternating the duration of your workouts on different days of the week. For instance, your workouts on Monday, Wednesday and Friday might be a bit longer than on Tuesday and Thursday.
- Depending on your exercise and training goals, consider breaking up your workout into 2 separate activities - 1 in the morning and 1 in the afternoon. This allows for a greater total time spent exercising per day while still adhering to the guidelines.
- Listen to what your body is telling you during and after your workout, as this can help to gauge whether your duration is acceptable.
- Remember to drink and eat if you decide to exercise longer than 30 minutes.
- Celebrate the fact that you are exercising, even if it is not for as long as you would like.

Additional Tips

Regardless of the intensity, frequency and duration of your exercise, there are some simple suggestions that can make your workouts more enjoyable and effective.

- ***Perform your workouts in cooler environments.*** This may include a well-ventilated gym, pool or the outdoors when the temperature is more favourable, such as mornings and evenings during the summer time. You may also find it helpful to complete your more challenging workouts in the pool, as it can help to keep a lower body temperature and heart rate while remaining comfortable. Refer to the chapter "Cross Training Your Way Through Pregnancy" for more tips.
- ***Stay hydrated during your workout.*** This will ensure that your working muscles and baby are the getting the nutrients they need. It will also help to regulate your temperature, minimize the risk of dehydration and the feeling of thirst. Although you tend to feel less thirsty when working out in cooler environments or temperatures, it is important to drink at regular intervals.

Refer to the chapter "Fuelling Your Pregnant Body" for more information.

- *Minimize your nausea.* If you experience a lot of nausea during your pregnancy, you might be prone to increased nausea during certain aerobic activities such as running. To help counterbalance this effect, try munching on something before, during or after your run. Good choices are carbohydrates like crackers, bagels and granola bars. If you do vomit, try sipping on fluids (as tolerable) to prevent dehydration.

- *Dress according to the weather.* During the summer, stay cool and avoid overheating. In the winter, dress in layers and wear material that wicks away sweat. Your body temperature rises faster during pregnancy and therefore, you may require fewer layers of clothes.

- *Invest in proper workout attire.* Investing in a high quality, supportive sports bra is a necessity to maximize comfort, provide better support and minimize sagging. Keep in mind that your breasts may get larger as your pregnancy progresses and you may want to stagger purchasing bras throughout your pregnancy to accommodate their growing size. You are also now more susceptible to yeast infections due to your higher levels of estrogen. Wearing cotton underwear and changing into dry clothes shortly after working out can help in avoiding a yeast infection.

Looking Fabulous While Working Out! Whoever suggested that you could simply borrow your husband's (larger) exercise garments certainly did not know about the Runningskirts Maternity Fitness Skirt designed in Canada. Not only are these skirts functional, they are extremely comfortable and make you feel and look great! Made from lightweight, quick-drying performance fabric, this maternity running and fitness skirt has a special built-in belly supporting waistband designed to go the distance...of all 3 trimesters. For further information or to place an order for the Maternity Fitness Skirt, go to www.runningskirts.com.

- *Wear a lower lumbar support belt.* Also referred to as the belly bra or pregnancy belt, this can be particularly helpful if you experience lower back pain during certain activities. Wearing the belt can help to offset the feeling of added weight on the belly that may be causing you to lean too far forward and putting excess strain on your lower back. However you should avoid wearing the belt at all times; doing so may weaken your core muscles further. To avoid becoming too dependent on the lumbar belt, it is important to maintain or begin a core strength program, as it will help alleviate your back pain, discomfort and prepare you for labour and delivery.

- *Alter your workout for comfort.* If your preferred choice of activity is not comfortable on a given day, try a different activity. Try your preferred activity again in a few days or weeks, as you may find that it is comfortable again. Otherwise, this may be a good time to experiment with other forms of exercises that will provide similar enjoyment.
- *Honour your body.* Your pre-pregnancy intense workout regime might have meant that you did not give yourself much downtime and workouts were typically done early in the morning or late at night. If at all possible, now is a good time to be gentler on your body, which may include scheduling your workouts at more decent times, enjoying some downtime during the day and permitting more days off.

Summary

Despite the availability of guidelines about exercise and pregnancy, there may be times when you have questions about exercising above and beyond the recommendations. We hope that you now have a better understanding of why the guidelines exist in the first place, as well as the potential risks associated with exercising beyond the recommended parameters. More importantly, we hope that the additional information presented in this chapter will help guide you in making your own decisions regarding how hard, how often and how long you will continue exercising during this 9-month period. If you are still unsure about your level of exercise, your best bet is to speak to someone who has worked with pregnant athletes. This can include your doctor or midwife, your coach or your personal trainer.

Chapter 7

PACING YOUR MIND

What if I find it difficult to scale back my workouts?
Is it normal to have mixed feelings about the timing of my pregnancy?
Will I have trouble coping if my pregnancy does not go as planned?

It's Not Just About the Physical Changes
Pregnancy is a period of time when your body goes through some pretty amazing transformations and it becomes increasingly important to listen to what it is telling you. In many cases, this may mean slowing down, decreasing your volume or intensity, or stopping exercise altogether. But listening to and acting upon what your body is telling you is not always easy - especially if your motivation to continue exercising and training remains strong. In fact, you may find yourself having to change the way that you *think and feel* about exercise during this 9-month period. Consider for a moment the following statements:

- Working out is an important aspect of your life.
- You are driven by the physical and the mental aspects of exercising.
- You have an inner drive that pushes you to train harder.
- You push your body to new limits and exercise through pain.
- You strive for personal bests in your performance.

In other words, there is more to exercising and training than physical exertion and improved performance; there is also a strong emotional component to it as well. As such, do not be surprised if you experience some reluctance and difficulty cutting back, both physically and emotionally, on your training during pregnancy and initially after giving birth. It can be difficult to scale back your workouts at first, especially if you are accustomed to pushing yourself through pain, pushing your body to the limit and always thinking about how to better your performance. Being an athlete is part of who you are and it can be hard to suddenly adjust your physical routines and beliefs about exercising.

Despite the need for physical and emotional adjustments during this period, most of the available information about exercise and pregnancy is focused solely on the *physical* considerations, such as your body's transformation or the recommended exercises and limitations. There is seldom any mention of the *emotional* considerations, such as:

- *I want to do what is best for my baby but I am not sure if I am ready to stop training hard.*
- *I feel like I "should" be exercising, even though my body is really tired.*
- *I worry about losing my competitive advantage.*
- *I am discouraged thinking about how hard it will be to regain my fitness after the baby is born.*
- *I was really looking forward to my upcoming race season and part of me is disappointed that I will not be able to finish it.*

Adjusting to the Change in Pace

Can you relate to any of the above statements? How do you deal with such mixed thoughts and emotions? How do you adjust your mental psyche and turn off your competitive juices? You will not find answers to these questions by researching clinical studies but you can find some words of wisdom from other moms that have experienced it for themselves. The following is a list of strategies that athletic moms have found helpful when dealing with the mental and emotional challenges of "letting go" and learning to better pace their mind.

Be Honest with Yourself

A first step is to acknowledge any uncertainty, discouragement or mixed feelings you may have toward your pregnancy and the impact that this may have on your training and racing season. Training, and possibly competing, has likely played a significant role in your life; it may not be easy to simply "let go" of your training and performance goals, especially if your pregnancy was unplanned. In fact, you may find that your mind (compared to your body) may need a bit more time to adjust to your pregnancy. "I could not relate initially to having a baby grow inside of me. It seemed surreal and I had a very hard time pulling back initially on the intensity," explains Kathie Howes, an Ironman finisher and mother of 2. Some women may also experience mixed emotions at first. Whereas they are happy to be pregnant, they are also a bit saddened that they are not able to finish their season and reap the results from their months of hard training. Such feelings or reactions are normal and you should not feel guilty about having them. Just as it is important to let your body adjust to the pregnancy, you need to give your mind some time to adjust, as well. Acknowledging your feelings upfront may help to facilitate this adjustment.

Appreciate What You Are Doing
It is easy to get hung up on what you are no longer doing, especially if you are accustomed to a particular routine or if you are surrounded by athletic friends and family. As difficult as this may be, avoid the temptation of comparing yourself to others or to your previous training regime. Instead, try to appreciate what you ARE doing - and take comfort in knowing that being active provides so many benefits for both you and your baby. Tania Jones, one of Canada's top marathoners and mother of 2, suggests keeping the *regime* of training, rather than the training per say. This might include maintaining a similar pre-pregnancy schedule but modifying the activity levels based on how you are feeling. For example, if your pre-pregnancy running schedule included a long run, a speed workout and a casual run, modify your program to include 3 runs a week but reduce the intensity and duration. If running becomes too uncomfortable, switch to a different sport and maintain a similar regime.

Find Other Ways to Stay Involved
Exercising at a lower volume and intensity does not mean that you need to hibernate and isolate yourself from your sport or your athletic friends. After all, participating in sports has many social benefits, including interacting with others and building off of each other's energy. Why toss away such benefits altogether? Consider joining your training partners on their light training day or join them for coffee or tea following their workout. Alternatively, you can find new

training partners who better match your pregnancy fitness level or join a prenatal fitness group. Morgan, a competitive swimmer and mother of 2, was not bothered so much by her slower swim times, but rather by the fact that she would have to move to a different swim lane, away from her friends. Her solution? She swam with fins, as this enabled her to swim fast while keeping her intensity low, alongside her friends. Another strategy is to participate in a sporting event solely for fun, instead of competing. You can still experience the sporting environment but in a much more enjoyable and relaxed manner. But be warned: this idea only works if you know that you can "hold back" and not let your competitive nature take over. Otherwise, leave your sporting gear at home and consider volunteering instead. You may find yourself appreciating the sport in a whole new way.

Remove Yourself From Temptation
You may find it necessary to distance yourself from all gadgets, routes and anything else that quantifies your performance, with possibly the exception of the heart rate monitor. You already know that your intensity and volume will inevitably decrease, so why constantly remind yourself of this only to get discouraged? If you know how long it would have taken to swim 100 meters prior to getting pregnant, avoid looking at the clock. If you know that it normally takes an hour to cycle your favourite bike route, find a new route and leave the cycling monitor at home. "I avoided looking at any numbers while exercising during my pregnancy. Rather, I chose to just listen to my body and go by feel; this was a refreshing mental break from the structure of always following my heart rate, power (watts), and speed," explains Danelle Kabush, professional Xterra athlete and mother of 2.

Have Patience
Sometimes, all it takes is a bit of time and patience for your emotional psyche to adjust to the change in pace. Once this happens, you may find that your goals and expectations toward exercising and fitness naturally begin to shift as your pregnancy progresses. For instance, although your initial intent may have been to maintain your pre-pregnancy fitness as much as possible, it is possible for your exercise goals to switch from "being as fit as possible" to "being as fit as necessary". In other words, the purpose of working out becomes more

about being strong and healthy to handle the physical and emotional demands of pregnancy and labour. Heather Lowe, a 2-time Ironman finisher and mother of 2, was accustomed to challenging workouts and pushing her body to the limit; however she had to learn to adjust mentally and let her body take the driver's seat. "I found it very frustrating that, despite my high motivation to exercise, my body sometimes had other plans," explains Lowe. "My frustration lessened once I decided to let my body win and gave myself permission to skip the workout on such a day. This took a bit of time, and required me to think about exercising in a new way."

My Story: The Power of a "Bump"

When I first became pregnant, I wanted to stay active and maintain as much fitness as possible, without putting the baby's health at risk. The thought of losing the fitness that I had gained over the past year of training, and then having to regain it all back after giving birth, was discouraging. I became even more discouraged when I saw how much my heart rate changed and how much slower I became in my 1st trimester. However, once several weeks passed and I developed a visible "belly bump", something changed emotionally for me. I no longer cared about the fitness that I was losing. Instead, I welcomed this "temporary break" and told myself that I would save my energy for my postpartum comeback. Who knew that this little "belly bump" could have such an effect on me and provide me with a new perspective?

Jennifer Faraone, co-author, competitive duathlete and runner, mother of 2

Believe in Yourself

Above all else, do not lose sight of the fact that this is a temporary adjustment. Reducing the volume and intensity of your training (or stopping it altogether), does not make you any less of an athlete. Believe that you will have the physical and mental toughness and dedication to return to the level of commitment and performance of your sport when the time is right for you and for your family. Learning to pace your mind will no doubt make you a better athlete in the long run as:

- You will be more adept at listening to your body.
- Both your body and mind will benefit from this form of rest.
- You will be increasing your chances of staying healthy and injury-free.
- You will be setting a good example for your little one about the importance of listening to your mind.

When Things Don't Go as Planned

Many women envision having the perfect healthy pregnancy – the nicely shaped and rounded belly, little or no morning sickness, minimal weight gain, that healthy "glow" and an overall sense of happiness. Although we would all love to have such an experience, not every pregnancy always goes as planned. Unfortunately, there is no crystal ball that can predict who will - and who will not - have an amazing pregnancy.

There are a variety of unplanned, unexpected and unwanted circumstances that may occur and greatly affect your overall pregnancy experience. At the more devastating end of the spectrum, approximately 15% of all known pregnancies will end in miscarriage. It is beyond the scope of this book to provide information regarding how to deal with such a painful and distressing situation. Should you have to face this difficult situation, and given the severity and intensity of emotions that usually accompanies a miscarriage, we strongly encourage you to speak to someone.

But even if you fall within the majority of women who carry their baby to term, there are other undesirable circumstances that may happen and can limit your ability to experience the pregnancy that you envisioned. Consider any of the following circumstances:

- You are extremely nauseous and have trouble keeping any food down.
- You have very little energy, which may be further worsened if you are caring for another child.
- You experience a significant amount of pain and discomfort on a daily basis.
- Your doctor has advised you to stop any form of exercise.

Making the Best of Things

My 2nd pregnancy did not go as expected. Unlike my 1st pregnancy, where I was able to run until my 3rd trimester, this time around I felt horrible when I ran. I also felt sick all the time and often experienced dizzy spells. What helped me cope was knowing that my pregnancy was temporary and that I would be back to running soon after the baby was born. I still needed a physical outlet of some sort - so on the days that I felt well enough I did walking hill repeats or stair repeats. It made me happy knowing that I persisted and stayed active and that this would benefit my baby.
Sharlene Cobain, competitive runner and mother of 2

- You have been placed on bed rest for the remainder of your pregnancy.

Any of the above scenarios can affect your overall pregnancy experience, your daily routine and your ability to remain active. Not surprisingly, you might experience feelings such as disappointment, frustration, anger or sadness. Thoughts like *"This is not what I envisioned"* or *"Why me?"* may enter your mind. So, how do you cope when your pregnancy does not go as planned? Although you may not realize it at first, your experience as an athlete might prove to be quite helpful. More specifically, the strategies that helped you cope with an injury or any setback that prevented you from training may also prove to be quite useful right now.

Acknowledge Your Feelings
As mentioned earlier, an important first step is to acknowledge the reality of the circumstances surrounding your pregnancy and recognize your own thoughts. Feelings of disappointment and sadness are normal reactions when your pregnancy is not what you envisioned. Similar to the frustration you may have felt when an injury forced you to take a pause from training, you may now be feeling similar emotions if you are placed on bed rest during your pregnancy. Not giving yourself permission to experience these emotions is unhealthy and could potentially lead to pent up emotions and compromise your ability to cope.

Speak to Someone
Talking to someone about how you feel can be a great outlet. It can also be an excellent way to explore your feelings and identify potential coping strategies. This person, which may include your partner, coach or friend, can lend an ear and may even be able to provide some helpful advice. Just as you might have found it advantageous or comforting to speak to another injured athlete who faced similar setbacks, you might find it helpful to speak to another pregnant athlete whose pregnancy did not go as planned. However, you may feel better speaking to someone outside your "inner circle" such as a professional counselor.

Write It Down
A journal can be a great asset to your training by keeping track of your progress and monitoring physical symptoms such as an upcoming cold

or the first signs of an injury. A journal can also be helpful to record any thoughts and emotions, such as anxiety, prior to an upcoming race. It is in this way that the journal can help you cope with undesired aspects of your pregnancy. The simple act of writing things down is a great way to explore your own thoughts and feelings, especially if there are some things that you would prefer to keep to yourself. Once you have written things down, it then becomes easier to identify steps or actions that can help channel your thoughts and emotions into more positive ones.

Think of the Bigger Picture

As hard as it might be, try not to lose sight of the bigger picture - that you are creating a beautiful and healthy baby. Remember that this is a temporary experience. These remaining months of your pregnancy *will* pass, you *will* feel better and you *will* gain control of your body once again. Although this may prove to be the most difficult of all the suggestions, it can greatly help to channel your energy toward more positive and productive thoughts.

I Can Do This

Getting pregnant in the first place was such a struggle for my husband and I. So when my doctor placed me on bed rest just 15 weeks into my pregnancy, I did not think twice about following his instructions. I was just so grateful to be pregnant, that I did not dwell on the fact that I was no longer able to run, let alone be on my feet for more than 10 minutes every 2 hours. I thought of other female athletes that continued to run strong after having kids and used them as my role models. Surely if other women did it, I could too! After gaining 70 lbs. during my pregnancy and giving birth to twins, I can proudly say that my racing times are pretty much back to where they left off!

Jennifer Drynan, competitive runner and mother of twin boys

Summary

Being pregnant is all about changes, the most obvious one being the physical changes that your body goes through. However, there are also some significant emotional challenges that you may experience, especially if your pregnancy does not go as planned. Although learning to pace your mind can be difficult at first, rest assured that this can be overcome with a few simple strategies including time, patience and confidence.

Chapter 8

CROSS TRAINING YOUR WAY THROUGH PREGNANCY

Why is cross training important right now?
Are some activities or sports better than others?
Are there certain considerations I should be aware of?

Choosing Your Activities
There are many reasons cross training is important for you as an athlete, such as improving your overall body strength, preventing or minimizing injuries and preventing boredom of always doing the same thing. Although these reasons continue to be relevant during your pregnancy, there are other benefits to cross training during this 9-month period. First of all, you may have chosen to, or have been advised to, discontinue participating in your preferred sport and are looking for alternative activities that will help maintain your fitness. Furthermore, some cross training activities designed specifically for pregnancy, such as prenatal yoga and Pilates, can be a great compliment to your sport as they emphasize relaxation, flexibility and full-body range of motion exercises. Such components could easily be lacking in your regular training program.

Regardless of your fitness level or chosen activities, the following suggestions can help get you started and tailor your workouts appropriately.

- *Start out slowly.* Begin exercising at a lower intensity when introducing a new activity during your pregnancy. Starting out more conservatively will give you a chance to see how your body responds to this new activity. You may be surprised by how your body feels after trying something new.

- ***Ease in/out of your workout.*** Complete a proper warm up and cool down for at least 5-10 minutes. A warm up ensures that your body has adequate time to adjust to the upcoming activity by mimicking the activity at a slower rate. The cool down allows your heart rate to come back down before stopping the activity, which should help prevent blood from pooling in the legs and causing any dizziness and/or fainting. Although this principle applies to all athletes, the need for an adequate warm up and cool down becomes increasingly important during pregnancy due to the added cardiovascular demands of pregnancy (as discussed in the chapter "The Pregnant Athlete's Body").

- ***Choose the timing of your activity.*** Consider waiting until you have finished the 1st trimester before introducing a new activity, as your body will have had the chance to get accustomed to the pregnancy. You may feel less tired and any morning sickness may have lessened or stopped altogether.

Take a Pass

Are there certain activities or sports that are best to avoid during your pregnancy? Definitely! The *PARmed-X for Pregnancy* recommends avoiding contact sports and sports/activities that may cause loss of balance or trauma to you or baby. These include:

Soccer	Basketball
Ice hockey	Roller blading
Horseback riding	Skiing/snow boarding
Sky diving	Scuba diving
Vigorous racket sports	
Hiking at altitudes above 8250 ft	

Cardiovascular Activities

There are many appropriate types of cardiovascular exercises to choose from, with only a few considerations, modifications or restrictions. Regardless of the cardiovascular activity, it is important to monitor your intensity. As discussed in the chapter "How Hard, How Often and How

Long", you can use any or a combination of the following methods to help determine and monitor appropriate exercise intensity: your modified heart rate training zone, Borg's Rating of Perceived Exertion (RPE), the talk test, your previous training history and a little common sense with respect to overdoing it.

Swimming

There are several reasons why swimming has been recognized as one of the safest forms of exercise during pregnancy. First of all, swimming is a non-weight bearing activity that most people find comfortable. As a result, many women find that they can swim right up until the end of their pregnancy. Second, swimming provides a natural resistance, which allows for a great challenging full-body workout. Third, it has been suggested that being in the pool allows you to stay cooler and therefore, more comfortable (assuming appropriate temperature of both the water and room). And finally, working out in the pool may also keep your exercise heart rate lower than working out on land.

There are, however, a few precautions to take when swimming. For starters, you may want to be a bit cautious when doing the breaststroke or using a kickboard in your 3rd trimester, as both may cause you to overarch and potentially strain your lower back. Similarly, kicks that are too deep or too wide may cause pelvic pain. If you are prone to heartburn, you might find that the horizontal position of swimming or flip turns may aggravate this condition. Finally, remember that swimming in a warmer pool puts you at greater risk of overheating and dehydration; if possible, stick to cooler pools, drink adequate amounts of fluid and monitor your core temperature.

Pool Running

Pool running, otherwise known as water running, works the body the same way that running does but without the impact, thereby lessening stress on your body. This, in combination with the cooler environment, will make you feel more comfortable while you exercise. For these reasons, pool running is a great alternative for doing workouts, including those that might be a bit more strenuous in nature.

It is important to maintain proper form when pool running. A good way to do this, especially if new to pool running, is to use some form of flotation device, such as an aqua belt or vest. The aqua belt or vest can help maintain a more upright posture and allow the arms and legs to produce a running motion, as opposed to treading water, which is the body's natural inclination. It may be possible to forego the belt as you develop proficiency, strength and can maintain proper form.

Proper form can be achieved by mimicking your running stride: keep your shoulders aligned with your hips, tuck your tailbone slightly underneath you and swing your arms at the shoulder joint in a forward and backward direction. Avoid leaning too far forward at the waist, as this can place strain on your lower back. Drive your knee up towards your waist and then let your foot come down beneath you. Relax your shoulders and avoid letting them round forward or creep toward your ears. If you are not sure whether you are using proper form, try finding a runner or an aquatic professional that has experience with water running and ask them to view your technique.

Cycling
Cycling is an amazing low impact cardiovascular activity for boosting your aerobic fitness and building strength in your legs. You can ride outdoors but you may want to consider switching to a stationary bike around your 4th or 5th month. This is approximately the time when you may experience a shift in your balance and your growing belly may start to get in the way of pedalling. Such changes may put you at greater risk of falling off the bike.

As you move into your 3rd trimester, consider switching to a recumbent bike (which looks more like you are sitting in a chair while pedaling) to relieve the pressure that upright cycling can place on the bladder, bowels, lungs and stomach. If you want to continue on the upright bike, it may be a good time to invest in a pair of padded shorts or padded seat cover to reduce any pressure on your backside or perineum region. You might also find it useful to raise the handlebar stem gradually as your belly grows and to adjust the seat to find the most comfortable position. Finally, staying in the saddle or seat while pedaling is a good idea if you are prone to knee pain or discomfort.

Walking
Walking has been suggested as a primary choice for physical activity among pregnant woman. It is one of the most convenient forms of cardiovascular exercise, as it only requires a good pair of running or walking shoes and can be done anywhere, anytime and by anyone.

However, a leisurely stroll in the park will not suffice if your goal is to maintain some of your fitness. To achieve such benefits, make sure you are walking at a brisk pace and can feel your heart rate increasing. To make it even more challenging, you can try walking on a hilly course, setting the treadmill on an incline or walking at a brisk pace with a light pair of weights in your hands. Regardless of which strategy you use, keep your shoulders aligned with your hips and avoid leaning forward at the waist.

Cross-Country Skiing

Cross-country skiing is another amazing low impact activity that works the entire body. As your sense of balance may shift throughout your pregnancy, it is best to stick to familiar trails and avoid challenging routes that can put you at risk of falling. Some experts suggest classic skiing (which is typically done in a track on groomed trails using a kick and glide motion) over skate skiing (which is done on wide opened-groomed trails using a V-step and glide motion), as the latter may require more balance and stamina.

Other Types of Cardiovascular Exercise Machines

Most cardiovascular exercise machines, such as the stair climber, elliptical trainer and cardio wave (which mimics the skating motion), are great cross training alternatives, as they provide a low impact aerobic workout that is comfortable and safe with a decreased risk of falling. Ensure you maintain proper form, as there is a tendency to rest your arms on the armrests or handles and to lean too far forward, placing strain on your lower back.

> **Getting Stronger**
>
> As it was getting more and more difficult to train on the bike throughout my pregnancy, I started to spend more time in the gym doing weights and core strength. Prior to this, I had never really focused on strength work. Looking back, I now realize that this likely enabled me to make a speedy recovery postpartum – including winning the World Masters Track Championship in cycling.
> *Susie Mitchell, competitive track cyclist and mother of 1*

Pilates

Pilates is a series of gentle, full-body, muscle strengthening, flexibility and range of motion exercises emphasizing the proper alignment of the entire body. Moira Merrithew, Executive Director, Education at Merrithew Health & Fitness™, explains that Pilates can provide many benefits to a pregnant woman including:

- Restoring and maintaining balance and proper postural alignment, which tends to shift during and after pregnancy.
- Promoting deeper breathing throughout the poses, which will further aid during labour.
- Stabilizing the lower back and pelvis region.

Although most exercises are safe to perform during pregnancy, there are a few restrictions that need to be respected, including avoiding lying on your back around the 16th week gestation (or earlier if you are starting to show), modifying abdominal exercises and limiting your range of movement with certain exercises. If you are trying Pilates for the first time, it is important to find a qualified instructor that has experience working with pregnant women.

Yoga

Many people agree that practicing prenatal yoga provides both physical benefits (e.g. added flexibility and strength) and emotional benefits (e.g. relaxation and reduced stress). Prenatal yoga can also help to prepare for the upcoming physical demands of labour and delivery by emphasizing breathing techniques and learning to engage your core muscles. It is, therefore, not surprising that many yoga studios and fitness centres are now offering prenatal yoga classes. For your convenience, we have also included a few simple poses at the end of the book in Appendix 3 "Yoga Poses for the Pregnant Athlete". These poses have been selected with the pregnant athlete in mind and can easily be done at home.

There is more to yoga than simply performing a series of poses. In fact, there can be a deeper and more internal experience that one can draw upon when practicing yoga. Monica Voss, Co-Owner and Director of the Esther Myers Yoga Studio, explains that the primary value of yoga lies in its ability to promote relaxation, internal awareness and the welcoming of one's intuitive nature. Below, Voss provides a brief explanation of this and touches on how it can benefit you during your pregnancy.

Meditation

Yoga can be a great form of meditation that allows you to develop and focus on your own internal awareness. Your experience as an athlete may mean that you are already in tune with your body but practicing yoga may lead to a much deeper and deliberate sense of awareness. As you continue to experience an abundance of emotional and physical changes during your pregnancy, yoga can allow your intuitive nature to surface and acknowledge your thoughts and feelings. Such reflection can help to calm your mind.

Breathing

Breathing, for the most part, is an unconscious activity. However, many athletes may not always appreciate or understand the significance and properties of relaxed breathing. Breathing from your stomach (also known as deep belly breathing) triggers a neurological response that promotes a sense of relaxation, whereas shallow breathing triggers the "fight or flight" response and is counterproductive to a sense of calmness. Learning how to breathe deeply in your belly can help you to deal with anxiety and stress in your everyday life, during your workouts and your upcoming labour. Practicing yoga helps to bring awareness to your breathing, creates time and space for relaxation and provides the opportunity to enhance your breathing patterns.

Relaxation

Whereas being fit may provide you with the stamina required for a potentially long labour, yoga can provide the much-needed relaxation. Such relaxation occurs on 2 levels: emotional and physical. As previously discussed, the meditative aspect of yoga, combined with the focused breathing, can help to calm your mind. At the same time, performing various poses and the simple act of touch can help to bring awareness and relaxation to your physical body. For instance, placing your hands on your rib cage and directing your attention to your breathing can help your muscles relax and decrease your heart rate.

But Don't Forget the Baby

Voss also emphasizes the added benefit that practicing yoga has for your relationship with your growing baby. Making time for relaxation, meditation and focused (but gentle) abdominal

> **Getting the Most from My Cross Training Workouts**
>
> I was able to ramp up my cross training workouts throughout my pregnancy, as I was no longer doing speed sessions on the track. I mostly did cardio machines and weights. I really enjoyed these cross training sessions. In addition to having a great workout, I found them to be mentally relaxing. I was not getting caught up in the details such as pace and distance, which inevitably happens whenever I run.
>
> *Seanna Robinson, competitive runner and mother of 2*

breathing gives you the opportunity to feel your little one inside your body, appreciate what is happening and connect emotionally with your baby.

Strength Training

You may have heard the old myth that lifting weights could create too much exertion and induce premature labour or miscarriage. Fortunately, we have come a long way and this myth has since been debunked. Although there are not many studies that have looked exclusively at strength training in pregnancy, there is agreement among experts that this activity can be safe and beneficial. The Canadian Society for Exercise Physiology (CSEP), for example, recommends strengthening exercises to help your body adjust to the pregnancy-related changes, thereby helping you perform everyday tasks more easily. For instance, rounded shoulders and lower back pain, which may be a result of postural imbalances during your pregnancy, can be combated by strengthening and lengthening the appropriate muscle groups. Furthermore, strength training may serve as an appropriate substitute for one of your cardiovascular workouts if, or when, your regular workouts become increasingly difficult or uncomfortable.

Developing Your Program

Most women with a healthy and uncomplicated pregnancy can adopt and/or maintain a strength training program; however, CSEP and the American College of Obstetricians and Gynecologists (ACOG) suggest waiting until your 2nd trimester to start this new activity. If strength training was part of your regime prior to pregnancy, keep in mind that the areas in which you will want to strengthen now may differ slightly. Although you might have focused primarily on the specific key muscles used in your sport, you will now want to ensure that you are also strengthening *all* major muscle groups, as they will be used to support your growing frame. We have provided the following guidelines to help get you started with your strength training program (or to modify your existing one):

- *Target all major muscle groups.* Your program should include exercises that strengthen all major muscle groups, including those of the upper and lower body and core. To keep things simple and manageable, we have categorized the muscles according to specific areas of the body, along with the primary muscles to strengthen within each area and suggested exercises (Table 8.0). We are not suggesting that you perform each of the following exercises in a single session. In fact, many of the suggested activities will strengthen more than one muscle at a time. Rather, we wanted to provide you with as many options as possible and give you the freedom to pick and choose the activities that work best for you. Just remember to choose at least 1 exercise per muscle group.

> **Learn to Talk the Talk**
>
> A **rep,** shortened for repetition, is the number of times you repeat a particular movement without taking any breaks. Once you have completed the targeted number of reps in a row, you have just completed 1 **set.** The total number of reps and sets that you perform varies depending on your exercise goals. For instance, performing a higher number of reps with lower weights for a given number of sets targets muscle endurance; a lower number of reps with higher weights for a given number of sets targets muscle strength. During pregnancy, an appropriate goal is to aim for 2 sets of a specific exercise, with 10-15 reps per set.

- *Lift the correct weight.* Aim to lift a weight that allows you to complete at least 10 but no more than 15 repetitions (reps) with maximum effort in proper form. Once you can perform 15 reps in good form, it is time to increase the weight for that particular exercise. For optimal results you must perform each set to the point of muscle fatigue (when your muscles are incapable of performing another rep in good form, even with maximum effort).

- *Aim for 2-3 sessions a week.* Although once a week could prove beneficial, research has shown that strength training 2-3 times per week is optimal for building strength. Plus, the more sessions you do, the faster you will see results. Space the sessions out 48 hours or more to ensure that your muscles have recovered.

- *Make it efficient.* If you are short on time, try alternating between upper and lower body parts on different days. For example, focus on your legs the first day, followed by exercises for your upper body the following day. This will help to cut down your workout time on a given day while ensuring that you are targeting all muscle groups in the week. With this approach, you can work out on consecutive days. Performing exercises at home, rather than at the gym, will also help to maximize your time. Many exercises can be done using your own body weight, exercise bands or a variety of items found in the home, such as water jugs filled with water.

- *Seek a professional.* If you are new to strength training, consider working with a personal trainer who has experience working with pregnant women. They can ensure you are doing the activities with proper form and can recommend modifications or restrictions.

Table 8.0 provides a list of suggested activities to help strengthen your pregnant body. Remember, it is not necessary to complete them all; rather feel free to pick and choose 1 or 2 from each muscle group. More detailed information can be found in Appendix 4 "Strengthening Exercises for the Pregnant Athlete", Appendix 8 "Core Strengthening Exercises" and the chapter "Your Silent Training Partner – Your Pelvic Floor Muscles".

Table 8.0: Strengthening Activities for the Pregnant Athlete

Muscle	Muscle Function	Suggested Exercises
LOWER BODY – Refer to Appendix 4		
Gluteus (buttock muscle)	Extends the hip and abducts the leg	• Step-ups • Squats • Reverse lunge and forward lunge
Quadriceps (thigh muscles)	Extends the knee	• Walking lunges • Squat plus woodchop
Hamstrings (back of thigh muscles)	Extends the hip and bends the knee	• Lying hamstring curl off ball
UPPER BODY – Refer to Appendix 4		
Trapezius, Rhomboids	Helps to move the shoulder blades	• Row with exercise tube • Rhomboid squeeze

(muscles around the shoulder blades)		
Latissimus Dorsi (back muscles)	Extension, adduction and medial rotation of the shoulder joint Plays a role with extension and lateral flexion of the lower torso	• Lat pull down • Bent over row on ball
Pectoralis Major (chest muscles)	Moves the upper arm into flexion, adduction and horizontal adduction	• Modified push-up • Regular push-up • Incline press off the ball • Chest flyes off the ball
Deltoids (main shoulder muscles)	Moves the arm overhead, in front, to the side and behind the body	• Lateral raise • Front raise • Shoulder press
Biceps (front arm muscles)	Flexes the elbow, helps to rotate the forearm	• Bicep curl with exercise tube • Hammer curl
Triceps (back arm muscles)	Extends the elbow	• Dips off a chair (or bench) • Overhead tricep extension seated on a ball
MUSCLES OF THE TRUNK – Refer to Appendix 8		
Erectors (back muscles along the spine)	Extends the spine	• Bridge • Bird dog • Plank
Rectus abdominus, internal oblique, external oblique, transversus abdominus	Forward flexes, laterally flexes and rotates the spine Stabilizes the spine	• Ball curls • Baby hugs • Plank

(abdominal muscles)		
PELVIC FLOOR MUSCLES – Refer to "Your Silent Training Partner – Your Pelvic Floor Muscles"		
Levator ani, Coccygeus	Provides support for the pelvic organs, bladder, intestine and uterus	• Pelvic floor exercises, also known as Kegels

Additional Considerations for Strength Training

Regardless of which strengthening exercise you perform, the following points are important:

- **Breath properly.** It is not uncommon to hold your breath while strength training. This usually occurs when you push yourself beyond your comfort zone. Although it is safe to go beyond your comfort zone, it is not a good idea to hold your breath because it could cause an unsafe increase in your blood pressure. As a good rule of thumb, be sure to exhale during your exertion.

- **Modify activities that put pressure on your wrists.** You may now be more susceptible to a condition known as carpal tunnel syndrome (CTS), in which the median nerve is compressed, causing wrist pain. During pregnancy, this compression may be caused by water retention or swelling in the wrist. If you experience any symptoms, it may be wise to avoid or modify activities that put stress on your wrists such as push-ups, tricep dips and some yoga poses including downward dog. You may find it helpful to contact a health care provider, such as a physiotherapist or chiropractor, to treat and alleviate your pain.

- **Modify exercises performed on your back.** Many sources, including CSEP and ACOG, suggest staying off your back while doing exercises by the 4th or 5th month (or sooner if you start to show), as you may feel light-headed and/or dizzy. That being said, some sources, including Dr. James Clapp, author of *Exercising Through Your Pregnancy*, believes that it is safe for you to perform exercises in the supine position provided that you are moving your legs and torso and do not feel dizzy. Supine exercises can also be modified by using a wedge, an inclined exercise bench or an exercise ball.

- ***Continue and modify core strengthening activities.*** It cannot be said enough that maintaining a strong core, including the abdominal and pelvic floor muscles, should happen before, during and after pregnancy. As such, we have dedicated the chapter "Your Strong And Powerful Core" to provide detailed information regarding how to perform core strengthening activities correctly. If you develop diastasis recti, a noticeable separation of your abdominal muscles (specifically rectus abdominis), see a qualified professional to learn how to modify some of the exercises. Doing the exercises incorrectly can lead to further separation of the abdominal muscles.

Summary

There are plenty of choices when it comes to selecting appropriate exercises activities during your pregnancy, including strength training, yoga, Pilates and numerous cardiovascular exercises. Selecting the right one is usually a matter of preference, safety and comfort. Equally important is the fact that you are remaining active while doing something that you enjoy.

Chapter 9

MONITORING THE HEALTH OF YOU AND YOUR BABY

If exercising is safe, why is it important to monitor the health of my baby and I?
Won't my doctor or midwife be doing the necessary checks?
Are there simple checks that I can do?

Looking Out for You and Your Baby

As detailed in previous chapters, most women can exercise throughout their pregnancy without causing harm to themselves or their babies. In fact, it is strongly encouraged that you continue to remain active, as opposed to stopping exercise altogether, if you are experiencing a healthy pregnancy. So, if exercising is considered safe, why are we devoting a chapter to the monitoring of the health of you and your baby? Quite simply, you are now moving into uncharted territory; you cannot always predict how your body will respond to a particular activity or to the added effect of multiple activities over time. Our intent is not to create any fear or anxiety. Rather, we are trying to show how a few simple checks can provide you (and others) with the reassurance that you are exercising in a safe manner.

It might have been easy to determine how much physical exertion your pre-pregnancy body could tolerate, how much rest you needed in between workouts or how much fluid you needed to consume during your workouts. However, these parameters become more unpredictable once you are pregnant. Following the recommended exercise guidelines discussed in previous chapters is a good start, but this alone may not be adequate. For instance, although you might be exercising within the recommended 30 minutes per day with an appropriate warm up and cool down, you are putting both yourself and your baby at risk if you routinely exercise in the middle of the hot and humid day without consuming adequate fluids.

Most of the monitoring methods we are suggesting will help flag if/when you are working out too much, require more rest in between workouts, need to take in additional fluids during your workout and so on. Taking a few simple preventative measures, such as working out in a well-ventilated environment and staying well hydrated, can affect how well your body can handle a particular workout, influence the timing and the quality of your next workout and ensure the well-being of you and your baby.

Your Prenatal Check Ups

In North America, most women with a low risk pregnancy will see their midwife or doctor every 4 weeks during the 1st and 2nd trimester. In the 3rd trimester, the visits are more often, typically once every 2 weeks until 36 weeks and then weekly until the baby is born. The purpose of these visits is to monitor the progression of your pregnancy and provide you with information to help keep you and your baby healthy. As a pregnant woman that exercises on a regular basis, should the frequency of your visits be any different? Not necessarily, unless you are training at a very intense or elite level. The amount and type of monitoring relates to your level of training - the more intense your training, the more monitoring is likely required.

Rest assured, we are not suggesting a long list of tests to be performed by you and/or your health care provider. After all, your doctor or midwife will be performing various checks throughout your entire pregnancy to monitor the well-being of you and your baby. In many cases, such tests are performed on a monthly basis and then more frequently in final weeks leading up to your due date. Keep in mind that if you are extremely active, your health care provider may want to monitor you more regularly. We also recommend that *you* take on an active role with the monitoring as it relates to your training, including overheating, dehydration, low blood sugar and the general well-being of you and your baby. As you shall soon read in Table 9.0, many of our suggested monitoring methods are quite simple, can be checked regularly and will allow you to make any changes to your training if needed.

Table 9.0: Suggested Monitoring Methods for the Pregnant Athlete

What to Monitor	Simple Checks
Body Temperature A temperature below 38.9°C (or 102.2°F) will help prevent overheating.	• Listening to your body is key; your body usually gives you plenty of signs and symptoms when you are starting to overheat. These may include shortness of breath, dizziness or nausea. • Ensure that you are working out in a well-ventilated space or when the weather is more favourable, such as first thing in the morning during the summer months. • Consider taking your temperature before and after a more challenging workout. • **More advanced:** A more accurate method is to use a rectal or vaginal thermometer.
Hydration Levels Being adequately hydrated allows your body to function optimally.	• Look at your urine following your workout to see if it is clear. If it is not, you may not have been drinking enough before and during your workout. • A second method is to weigh yourself before and after your workout to ensure that your post-workout weight does not drop more than 2%. • **More advanced:** Tests can be performed to measure your hematocrit or plasma protein concentrations, as low levels could be signs of dehydration.
Blood Glucose Glucose stores (sugar levels) provide the necessary energy to function.	• Ensure that you have adequate nutrition and fluid intake before, during and after you exercise, as this is where your body gets its glucose. • Watch for sudden feelings of shakiness, light-headedness, fatigue or anxiety; these could be signs of low blood sugar. • **Note:** This is not to be confused with gestational diabetes, which is when you have higher than normal blood glucose levels.

Iron Stores Your pregnant body now requires additional iron.	• Several studies have found that many female athletes struggle to keep their iron levels up. Taking prenatal supplements with a high level of iron and eating iron-rich food sources will help to promote adequate iron stores. • Talk to your doctor if you notice any of the following: feeling more tired, weak and dizzy, pale skin, rapid heartbeat, heart palpitations, shortness of breath or trouble concentrating. • **More advanced:** Blood tests can be performed to check your hemoglobin, hematocrit, and ferritin levels several times throughout your pregnancy.
Your Well-Being Feeling physically, mentally and emotionally strong ensures a happy, healthy pregnancy.	• Pay attention to how you feel during your workouts and look for noticeable differences between similar workouts. • Keep an eye on your energy levels throughout the day, as well as your overall mood. • A journal may be helpful for keeping track of things and answering self-evaluation questions such as: Are your workouts feeling like they are a lot harder than they were a few days ago? Are you constantly feeling very sluggish in your workouts? Are you run-down and needing to rest more often? Are you no longer motivated to exercise? These could be signs that you are doing too much and you may want to consider taking a few days of rest.
Baby's Well-Being Your baby moves in a typical pattern during your pregnancy.	• Ensure that your baby continues to demonstrate his/her typical movement patterns before and 20-30 minutes after your workout. • Any mild uterine contractions that you feel while exercising should diminish quickly once you have stopped. Speak to your doctor or midwife if you have any concerns.

	• **Note:** Your doctor or midwife will be paying attention to your baby's health (heart rate and growth) during your prenatal visits.

Know When to Stop

In addition to the above monitoring methods, keep in mind that there are other symptoms you should always be on the alert for *during or after you exercise*, as described in the chapter "To Train or Not To Train". You should stop exercising immediately and seek medical attention if you experience any of the following: excessive shortness of breath, chest pain, light-headedness, painful uterine contractions, leakage of amniotic fluid or vaginal bleeding.

Summary

Participating in the regular monitoring of the health of you and your baby during and after your workouts will help to ensure that you are exercising at an appropriate level and taking the necessary preventative measures. Be sure to keep your health care provider in the loop with your findings and speak to him/her if you have questions or concerns.

Monitoring the Pregnant Athlete

Dr. Julia Alleyne, a sport and exercise physician, encourages respecting the guidelines when training during pregnancy. However, if a particular athlete feels the need to exercise outside the guidelines, she suggests starting with one element first, such as frequency, intensity, time or type of exercise. It then becomes easier to evaluate how the body responds to such an activity. Alleyne also stresses the importance of self-monitoring on a regular basis and as needed, frequent monitoring by their health care provider. Self-monitoring can include tracking pain and discomfort, the colour of urine, diet and sleep patterns. As required, health care providers can easily administer a fetal ultrasound, monitor urine and fluid levels, pain or discomfort, diet and sleep patterns. This monitoring will help to determine how hard the athlete is exercising and how she may progress. If her body responds favourably, she can bump up her training. Otherwise, she should revisit the guidelines and workout at a more comfortable level for the time being.

Chapter 10

GETTING SIDELINED

Do I have a higher risk of injury if I exercise throughout my pregnancy?
What are the most common injuries, conditions and symptoms?
What can I do if I get injured?

Your Risk of Injury

As a woman who exercises on a regular basis, you likely know first-hand that the majority of athletes experience some form of sports-related injury at some point or another. Common causes include overtraining, inadequate recovery between workouts and poor biomechanics, such as muscle imbalances. Unfortunately, your risk of injury does not magically disappear once you are pregnant, even if you have reduced the volume and intensity of your training. The fact of the matter is that sports-related injuries may be somewhat inevitable, despite your best intentions to avoid them from happening in the first place. Furthermore, some experts suggest that you may *now* have an increased risk of injury because of the numerous changes that your pregnant body is experiencing, including postural changes and hormonal

Do Pregnant Women Get Injured More?

Some experts suggest that pregnant women have a higher risk of injury as a result of the changes to their bodies. To investigate this claim, a 2010 study in North Carolina looked at how often pregnant women were injured as a result of exercising. Their results are encouraging; they found that the rate of exercise-related injury during pregnancy was an estimated 4.1 injuries per 1,000 hours of exercise - which is less than 1%! Furthermore, only 1/3 of the reported injuries actually took place *during* exercise. The most common type of injury was bruising or scraping, followed by strains and sprains. The take-away message? Keep exercising and do not let the fear of getting injured stop you.

fluctuations (specifically relaxin, which is responsible for the increased joint laxity during your pregnancy). Dr. Jennifer Wise, a chiropractor and co-founder of Thrive Natural Family Health, and who commonly treats women during pregnancy and the postpartum period, explains the importance of listening to one's body through pregnancy and adjusting their expectations. "I see a lot of women who expect the same performance from their bodies once they are pregnant. There are many structural changes in the body that could make the same activity more difficult, unsafe and may lead to an injury."

However, before getting too discouraged, take notice of the following: although the *theory* is that you may be more susceptible to injury during your pregnancy, no studies have actually found this to be the case. Nevertheless, it is still a good idea to continue to train wisely and apply some common sense, including gradually increasing your activity levels, stopping any activity when it does not feel right and giving your body ample time to rest.

Our intent with this chapter is not to describe all of the different types of injuries, conditions or nagging symptoms that you could potentially encounter during this 9-month period; that would be a very long list! Rather, we have chosen to focus on a select few that are perhaps more relevant to you as a pregnant athlete and could potentially interfere with your ability to exercise. Whether you encounter an example listed below or another injury altogether, the take away message is the same: listen to what your body is telling you, modify or stop the activity that is causing your symptoms and seek help from a qualified professional if the symptoms do not recede.

Round Ligament Pain

Round ligament pain is quite common during pregnancy and occurs more frequently in the 2nd trimester. The round ligament is one of several ligaments that surrounds and supports your growing uterus and connects it to your groin. As your baby (and uterus) grows, your ligament stretches, sometimes to the point where the ligament becomes strained. Certain exercises or movements that cause the ligaments to stretch and contract quickly, such as sneezing, coughing, going from sitting to standing quickly or fast running may cause pain. Classic symptoms may include a brief sharp pain or jabbing feeling in either the lower belly or groin area and can be felt on one or both sides. Fortunately, the pain should only last a few seconds.

The best treatment is to reduce the intensity of the activity that is causing the pain; if that does not cause the symptoms to lessen, you may want to consider stopping the activity temporarily. Additionally, you can try resting, taking a warm bath, avoiding sudden sharp movements and possibly taking pain-reducing medication (as prescribed by your doctor). Flexing your hips when sneezing, bringing your knees toward your stomach or lying on your side with a pillow under your belly and between your legs may help to relieve some of the discomfort. A chiropractor, physiotherapist or massage therapist who has experience treating pregnant athletes might be able to provide some relief with soft tissue therapy, such as the Active Release Technique (ART), Graston Technique or Swedish massage. Finally, consider seeing your doctor if the symptoms have not decreased after a few days.

> **My Story: Learning the Hard Way**
> I did a 5K "fun" race when I was about 4 months pregnant. Even though I had every intention of running easy, my enthusiasm took over and I ran harder than I should have. The next morning, while trying to get out of bed, I felt a sharp jabbing pain in my lower abdomen, a classic sign of round ligament pain. My chiropractor suggested that I might have strained the ligament by running too fast the previous day. Fortunately the pain soon passed and I made sure to tone it down a bit on my next few runs!
> *Jennifer Faraone, co-author, competitive duathlete and runner, mother of 2*

Low Back Pain

Low back pain during pregnancy is also fairly common. It is an all-encompassing term often used to describe a variety of symptoms. There are actually 2 main types of pregnancy-related low back pain —low back pain itself and pelvic girdle pain (described next).

Low back pain can be felt between your last rib and the top of your hips. It has been reported that close to 90% of women suffer from some form of low back pain during their pregnancy and almost 1/3 report that their first episode of low back pain occurred during their pregnancy. Approximately 10-25% of women rate their low back pain as moderate to disabling. Unfortunately, the exact reason for such pain is not well understood. A number of explanations have been suggested, such as weight gain, a shift in the centre of gravity, weakness of abdominal muscles and hormonal fluctuations but, to date, none have been proven. It is likely a combination of these explanations that is the true culprit.

Low back pain during pregnancy has been described as dull, causing movement to be restricted due to the pain and tightness of certain muscles in the lower back – especially the erectors that run along either side of the spine. Given how common low back pain is during pregnancy, it is not surprising that it may be aggravated by certain activities like running or cycling. If you are not able to relieve your back pain on your own and/ or if the pain radiates down into your legs, speak to your doctor or a qualified professional for additional help. A chiropractor, physiotherapist or massage therapist can help relieve some of the muscle tightness, and suggest core strengthening exercises and low back stretches.

Pelvic Girdle Pain

The pelvic girdle, which is comprised of the 2 hip bones (iliac crest) and the sacrum, is held in place by a network of connective tissue and ligaments. During pregnancy, the ligaments and connective tissue soften as a result of an increase in the hormone relaxin, thereby causing the joints to be more mobile, possibly misaligned and irritated.

Pelvic girdle pain, also known as pelvic pain or symphysis pubis pain, can be experienced anywhere between the hip bones and the end of the buttocks. Typically this pain can be felt either at the front of the pelvis (an area known as the symphysis pubis) or on one or both sides of your sacro-iliac joints (where your sacrum and hip bones meet) and in very severe cases, you may experience pain in all 3 areas. The pain may come and

My Bruised Ego (or Placenta!)

I was cycling with a training partner early in my pregnancy. Although my intent was to ride at a moderate pace, I decided to cycle harder when my training partner increased their intensity. After all, I was feeling good and was confident that my body could handle it. Perhaps I was mistaken. Although I finished the ride without experiencing any symptoms, my next ultrasound showed that I had bruised my placenta. I am not sure that the biking session was the cause, as even implantation (of the fertilized egg) can lead to bruising. Nevertheless, my doctor instructed me to modify my workouts until the bruise disappeared. Because of the bruise, I decided to play it safe and take precautions to make sure my hard training wasn't either causing it or preventing it from healing.

Tara Norton, professional triathlete and mother of 1

go and has been described as stabbing, shooting, dull or burning and may radiate down the back of your thigh(s). Symptoms can be aggravated when walking, climbing stairs, standing on one leg or turning over in bed.

Close to 20% of women experience PGP during their pregnancy and for some, the symptoms can extend into the postpartum period. Symptoms may emerge as early as the 1st trimester. However, it is more common in the middle of your pregnancy and may worsen with subsequent pregnancies. Since PGP can persist throughout your entire pregnancy (and postpartum) you may want to seek help before it worsens. An experienced physiotherapist, chiropractor or osteopath can help to relieve or ease your pain, improve muscle function, correct stiffness and/ or improve your pelvic joint position. They may also suggest exercises to strengthen your pelvic floor, stomach, back and hip muscles, as well as certain positions to assist with labour and delivery. Performing exercises in the water (such as swimming or pool running) or wearing a lower lumbar support belt may provide some relief.

Plantar Fasciitis
A common injury among athletes, especially runners, plantar fasciitis is an inflammation of the thick fibrous band of tissue that runs along the bottom of your foot. A classic symptom is pain in your heel when you first step out of bed in the morning. The pain normally lessens as your foot limbers up; however, it may return after long periods of standing, after getting up from a seated position or after certain activities that place a lot of stress on your heel and surrounding tissues.

Unfortunately, the research regarding pregnancy and foot pain is scarce. In a study by Vullo and colleagues (1996), it was found that just over 1/3 of their sample suffered from some form of foot pain during pregnancy, most often in the 2nd or 3rd trimester. Although these researchers did not provide an explanation of the cause of the pain, Anna Maria Infante, a chiropodist (foot specialist) at Bolton Family Foot Care, explains that pregnant women have an increased risk of developing this condition for several reasons – including the increased level of the hormone relaxin and the weight gain that causes the arches in your feet to flatten or collapse inwards. This collapsing or flattening of the arch may also cause the middle of your foot to roll in with each step, otherwise known as over-pronation.

Treatment may include resting, icing, stretching (including calf and hamstring muscles), taping, massaging and possibly, taking a break from certain weight bearing and high impact sports like running. If you are not able to relieve these symptoms on your own, seek help from a qualified health professional such as a physiotherapist, chiropodist/podiatrist or chiropractor to be fitted for an orthotic. Hasinah Shaqiq, a chiropodist at the MedCan Clinic, cautions that the foot (or arch) may not necessarily return to normal following pregnancy and further reinforces treating the foot early, to minimize changes in the foot and lessen the symptoms.

Knee Pain

Vladutiu et al. (2010) found that almost 25% of women experienced knee pain at some point in their pregnancy. The exact cause for such pain is not always known but there are several explanations, including an increase of the hormone relaxin, weight gain, changes in your gait pattern, a shift in your centre of gravity and an increased amount of time spent in the side-lying position. Regardless of the cause, the end result is often misalignment of the patella (kneecap) causing a grinding of the bones behind your knee and/or pain behind and surrounding the kneecap.

Consider seeing a qualified health professional, such as a physiotherapist or sports medicine physician, to help identify the cause of your pain. Treatment will likely involve stretching and strengthening

Your Changing Running Gait

Although you may not be aware of it, the way that you run (otherwise known as your running form or gait) might slowly change as your pregnancy progresses. You can blame it on the physical and hormonal changes taking place during this time: the relaxing of your joints, the shift in your centre of gravity, the increased curvature of your spine and the over-pronation of your feet. Such changes may place you at greater risk for overall pain and/or injury, as your feet are now striking the ground differently and your knees and hips are taking on new stresses.

What should you do? Begin by simply being aware of these changes and perhaps erring on the side of caution by keeping your running mileage at a reasonable level. Trying to "correct" your new running gait or forcing your body to respond in a certain way, could potentially lead to more problems over time. Once you are ready to start increasing your mileage after the baby is born, it may be a good idea to have your running gait looked at by a qualified professional at a sports clinic and if necessary, gradually work on improving your form.

the primary muscle groups including the hips, quadriceps and hamstrings. Modification of certain activities or exercises may also be required.

Summary
Although we have reviewed just a few of the more common injuries or discomforts that you could potentially encounter throughout your pregnancy, there may be others. Listening to your body and quickly acting on any signs and symptoms will help keep you healthy and active. Seeing your doctor or receiving treatment by a qualified health care professional may be necessary if your symptoms do not lessen after a few days.

Chapter 11

FUELLING YOUR PREGNANT BODY

Will my pre-pregnancy diet be suitable to meet the needs of both my baby and I?
Do I need to eat more if I exercise frequently?
Do I need to make further changes to what I eat and drink during my workouts?

The Pregnant Athlete's Diet

As an athlete, it is likely you have already adopted proper eating habits, including a food plan based on fruits and vegetables, whole grains, proteins, healthy fats and calcium-rich foods. Furthermore, you may also be following some of the more common principles of healthy eating, such as:

- Eating a combination of 45-65% of calories from carbohydrates, 10-35% from protein and 20-35% from dietary fats (comprised primarily of mono/polyunsaturated fats and essential fatty acids).
- Eating smaller and more frequent meals rather than 3 large meals.
- Enjoying all foods in moderation (including the occasional indulgence).

If so, you will be happy to know that your diet does not need to change significantly now that you are pregnant, as the diet of an athlete and that of a pregnant woman are very similar. While we could spend the next several pages detailing the typical diet for an athlete or a pregnant woman, such information is already well covered in countless books and other trustworthy resources. Rather, we have chosen to focus this chapter on some of the *additional considerations* for the pregnant athlete, such as the added calories that may be required and the type of nutrients to be consumed (and when) given your active lifestyle. As you will soon read, there are a few suggestions that can contribute toward more enjoyable and satisfying workouts while providing you with the reassurance that you are properly fuelling yourself and your baby throughout the day. Finally, keep in mind that specific nutritional considerations may vary slightly according to the individual and her particular sport. Speaking with a registered dietitian can further help to determine your exact needs.

> **Basic Staples of a Pregnant Woman's Diet**
>
> Proper nutrition during pregnancy plays a key role in the growth and development of your baby, while ensuring you also meet the nutritional demands of your ever-changing body. A typical diet for the average pregnant woman may include the following:
>
> - Approximately 350-450 extra calories per day in the 2nd and 3rd trimesters; more so if you are active.
> - 6-11 servings of breads and grains, 2-4 servings of fruit, 4 or more servings of vegetables, 4 servings of dairy products and 3 servings from protein sources.
> - A selection of foods high in fibre.
> - A prenatal multivitamin supplement with a higher amount of iron and folic acid.
> - Limiting (or avoiding) caffeine intake to 200-300mg.
>
> Refer to Appendix 5 *My Food Guide Servings Tracker* developed by Health Canada for more information.

Eat *Slightly* More

Are you thinking that pregnancy gives you a free pass to eat as much as you like? Hold on before eating that tub of ice cream. Gone are the days where a pregnant woman is eating for two. Angela Dufour, performance dietitian with the Canadian Sports Centre Atlantic, advises that the average pregnant woman needs to maintain her balanced and adequate pre- pregnancy diet during her 1st trimester and add ~350-450 extra calories per day during her 2nd and 3rd trimesters. These additional calories are needed to meet the demands of your growing baby. This increase could equal an extra 2-3 food group servings per day, like 5 whole grain crackers topped with 50g cheese or ¾ cup low fat yogurt with ½ cup berries and ¼ cup granola. But here lies the exception: an active pregnant woman that exercises regularly, such as 3-4 times a week at moderate intensity, will need to consume *even more* calories. How much more? That depends on the individual and her exercise type, duration and intensity.

Although there are few studies, if any, which focus on nutritional requirements for the pregnant athlete, there are some straightforward guidelines that can help determine your needs. A simple approach is to make sure that you are eating and drinking on a regular basis and perhaps a bit more on the days

My Story: Treating Myself

Although I did not monitor my calorie intake during my pregnancy, I simply made sure that I ate a bit more on the days I exercised or when I was feeling hungry. I must confess, however, that I did enjoy being slightly less disciplined with my eating habits and savouring fresh baked scones more frequently!

Jennifer Faraone, co-author, competitive duathlete and runner, mother of 2

that you are working out, to ensure you have replaced the calories spent while exercising. Although it can be a bit challenging to calculate this calorie expenditure, it is helpful for you to understand how many calories you are burning during various forms of exercise. To give you an idea, we have provided the table below that outlines the calories burned for the non-pregnant athlete (Table 11.0).

Table 11.0: Calories Burned During Different Types of Exercise for the Non-Pregnant Athlete

Activity (1 hour duration)	Weight of Person and Calories Burned		
	160 lbs (73 kg)	200 lbs (91 kg)	240 lbs (109 kg)
Aerobics, high impact	533	664	796
Aerobics, water	402	501	600
Backpacking	511	637	763
Bicycling, <10 mph	292	364	436
Canoeing	256	319	382
Golfing, carrying clubs	314	391	469
Hiking	438	546	654
Rowing, stationary	438	546	654
Running, 8 mph	861	1,074	1,286

Skiing, cross-country	496	619	741
Stair treadmill	657	819	981
Strength training	365	455	545
Swimming, laps	423	528	632
Tennis, singles	584	728	872
Walking, 3.5 mph	314	391	469

Source: Mayo Clinic Staff [Internet]. Rochester: Mayo Foundation for Medical Education and Research. Exercise for weight loss. c1998-2014 [last updated unknown; cited Jan 2014]; [about 1 screen]. Available from: http://www.mayoclinic.org/healthy-living/weight-loss/in-depth/exercise/ art-20050999.

Alexis Williams, dietitian for Loblaws Stores, further suggests that the number of calories burned will be a little higher in your 2nd and 3rd trimester. We are not indicating that you must replace every single calorie. However, eating only when you feel hungry can be a bit risky, especially if you tend to feel nauseous on a regular basis. In such a case, you may want to consider eating some form of easily digestible, higher calorie snacks such as a smoothie or a prenatal meal replacement beverage. Finally, staying within the recommended weight gain guidelines (as discussed in the chapter "The Pregnant Athlete's Body") can provide further reassurance that you are consuming enough calories.

Eat More of the Right Food Sources

Eating a well-balanced diet is important for both athletes and pregnant women. As a pregnant athlete, however, you may want to pay a bit more attention to your intake of the following 3 nutrients: protein, carbohydrates and iron. This is because your body now has a double-duty reliance of these food sources in order to meet the demands of your athletic pursuits, combined with your growing baby.

Protein

As an athlete, your body uses protein to repair the microscopic tears in your muscles following a hard workout. As a pregnant woman, your body uses protein to help your baby's growth and to form important organs like the brain. Not surprisingly, your body's increasing need for protein rises most in the 2nd and 3rd trimesters, as this is when your baby's growth is fastest, requiring additional nutrients. Although the general recommendation is to consume an additional 10-25g of protein during pregnancy, some clinicians have cautioned that many North American women may already consume enough protein in their diet. As an athlete, you may want to review your protein intake and consider aiming for the upper range of additional protein (i.e. 25g), if you are not already meeting this amount. This will ensure that your recovery needs are met; otherwise, the protein directed to your recovery may be limited, as it will be directed to meet the needs of your baby first, thereby reducing any amount left over to heal your tired muscles.

Carbohydrates
Your active body (including your heart, brain and muscles) thrives on carbohydrates, the key fuel source for exercise, especially during prolonged continuous or high intensity exercise. Not surprisingly, this nutrient also serves as the primary fuel source for your growing baby. Therefore, your body's demand for this source will also increase during the 2nd and 3rd trimester. Not consuming enough carbohydrates can limit the growth of your baby. There is also some evidence that pregnant women may use carbohydrates at a greater rate both at rest and during exercise than non-pregnant women, thereby supporting the importance of consuming this nutrient regularly throughout the day, not just before/during/after exercise.

If you were eating a well-balanced diet prior to getting pregnant, you may not need to make any drastic changes. That being said, Dufour, who has also written *PowerFuel Food: Planning Meals for Maximum Performance,* cautions that the majority of female athletes she works with tend to under-consume their calorie intake during regular training. She therefore suggests making sure that you, an active pregnant woman, consume a diet that is comprised of approximately 45-65% (or more) carbohydrates and that additional carbohydrates are consumed during prolonged workouts over 30-60 minutes (depending on the activity) and immediately following your workout (ideally with some protein). An exception is if you have gestational diabetes, as your carbohydrate intake may need to be slightly lower (e.g. 40-50%). Timing your meal and snacks appropriately with the inclusion of protein will help stabilize the blood sugars and ensure there are enough carbohydrates to support your activity.

Iron

Your athletic body uses iron to make hemoglobin - the rich, red blood cells that carry oxygen from your lungs to your muscles. Studies have shown that iron deficiency is a common problem for athletes, in particular endurance athletes. Vegans, or anyone else who restricts their meat intake, make be at risk as well. During pregnancy, your iron requirements rise even more in response to an increase in your blood volume and your growing baby and placenta. It is not uncommon for women (athletic or not) to start their pregnancy with insufficient stores of iron. It is therefore recommended that you take a prenatal multivitamin that has a higher dose of iron - usually 27mg. Too much iron is just as bad as too little iron, so speak with your doctor before taking any additional supplementation past a multivitamin. Better yet, ask your doctor or midwife to monitor your iron throughout your pregnancy, especially if you have a history of low iron or anemia. This can be done with a simple blood test to check your hemoglobin (the molecules that carry the iron) and ferritin (your iron stores or reserves) levels.

Drink Up

The amount of fluids that your body needs to stay properly hydrated increases once you are pregnant. Not surprisingly, the more you sweat during exercise, the more fluid you will require. Ensuring that you are drinking regularly during the day, carrying a water bottle with you at all times, eating juicy fruits, avoiding feeling thirsty and making a conscious effort to drink more before, during and after you exercise are all ways of staying hydrated.

Not sure if you are hydrating enough? The most basic (and simple) way of checking is to look at your urine. Clear or pale yellow urine means that you are properly hydrated. A darker yellow means you need to drink more. A word of caution: certain types of prenatal multivitamin may cause a slight discolouration of your urine, making this method less accurate. A more advanced method is to compare your weight pre and post workout, ensuring you have not lost more than 2% of your body mass.

Fuelling Your Workouts

Consuming adequate calories during your workouts is even more important now that you are pregnant, as your body is providing the fuel for both you and your baby. So, if you were not attentive to your calorie intake pre- pregnancy, now is a perfect time to start! According to Jennifer Sygo, dietitian at Cleveland Clinic Canada, it may not be necessary to consume additional fluids and carbohydrates if you exercise for less than 30 minutes, provided that you have been eating and drinking 1-2 hours beforehand. But if you are planning on exercising for longer or if it is a hot or humid day, it is important that you refuel throughout your workout.

The same types of supplements or sport products that you consumed prior to getting pregnant, such as gels, chews and bars, are probably safe to continue using. However, you may want to pay extra attention to the amount of caffeine (if any) included in each product. Gel packs are perhaps the most common product with added caffeine but different types of chews may contain caffeine as well. Furthermore, it is best to consume a sports drink as opposed to an energy drink that may contain caffeine or guarana (a fruit with higher caffeine content than coffee). Finally, consider taking a pass on any performance-enhancing products (also known as an ergogenic sports supplement), even if you were consuming them prior to pregnancy. There is limited, if any, research conducted on pregnant athletes and this type of supplement's long term effects on mother and child.

> **Give Yourself a Boost**
>
> Stocking up on foods rich in vitamin C, such as most fruits and veggies, is a great idea for pregnant athletes, recommends Lianne Phillipson-Webb, founder and nutritionist of Sprout Right. Consuming a high amount of vitamin C will help boost your immune system, which otherwise can be slightly suppressed during pregnancy and can make you more vulnerable to viral infections such as coughs, colds and flu. Phillipson-Webb recommends an upper limit of 2000mg per day for most of your pregnancy and 1000mg in your last month. This recommendation becomes increasingly important for pregnant women that participate in prolonged bouts of strenuous exercise, which can also suppress your immune system. If you are starting to feel run down or feel a cold coming on, consider skipping the workout and treating yourself to a nice warm bowl of chicken soup instead.

Additional Support

Although the information mentioned above is relatively straightforward, ensuring the proper intake of food and fluids can be challenging, especially if:

- You are feeling nauseous and have trouble keeping food down.
- Many foods are "turning you off."
- You are not gaining enough weight.
- You are gaining too much weight.

If any of the above applies to you, take charge and find a registered dietitian that has experience working with pregnant athletes. They can quickly provide you with a wealth of information and practical strategies.

Summary

Assuming you previously ate a well-balanced diet and replenished adequately during and after your workouts, you will be happy to know that your diet during your pregnancy should, more or less, stay the same with just a few modifications. Otherwise, now is a perfect time to start paying attention! Some of the simple suggestions we recommend include increasing your daily calorie intake, eating adequate quantities of foods/fluids that are high in carbohydrates and protein, keeping your iron stores elevated, staying well-hydrated, and consuming adequate fluids and food during/after your workouts. An experienced registered dietitian can also provide specific recommendations tailored to your individual needs.

Chapter 12

PREPARING FOR THE BIG EVENT

What can I expect during childbirth?
Will being fit make my labour easier?
What can I do to better prepare myself for labour?

3...2...1...Go!

After 9 months of anticipation, the big day has finally arrived! Although you may have read several books on the topic or heard numerous birthing stories from other moms, you cannot help but wonder *what is it really like?* Many women say that it is hard to give an accurate description of what it is like to give birth. Every woman's birthing experience is unique and no amount of planning and

> **Strange but True Stories from the Birthing Room**
>
> Although there is a typical sequence of events that happens during labour, there is always room for surprises in the delivery room. Jessica Zelinka, a Canadian Olympic heptathlete, 100m hurdler and mother of 1, strained her husband's bicep while pushing during an intense contraction. Fiona Whitby, a professional triathlete and mother of 1, pushed so hard while trying to expel her placenta, that it literally flew across the room! How's that for demonstrating female strength!

preparation can forecast what your labour will be like. How long the labour will last, how intense the pain will be and what types of medical intervention may be necessary, are all unknown. What is known, however, is the typical pattern of labour and the process required for the baby to make its way down the birthing canal and out into the world (Table 12.0). But what else do we know about labour and delivery? Can your active lifestyle and commitment to your sport influence childbirth? Will it make it easier? Faster? Less painful?

Jennifer Faraone & Dr. Carol Ann Weis

Table 12.0: Typical Progression of an Uncomplicated Labour and Delivery

Stage*	Description	What You May Feel	How to Cope
#1 Early Labour & Active Labour	Uterus starts to contract or tighten; cervix thins out and begins to dilate from 0-10cm. Stage is further broken down into: Early: cervix dilates to 3cm. Active: cervix dilates to 10cm. Transition: last part of active labour, you are "transitioning" to the pushing phase of labour.	Early: Mild contractions at first and then beginning to intensify. Active: More intense contractions, lasting 60-90 seconds and 3-4 minutes apart. Transition: More painful and frequent contractions, about 2-3 minutes apart, lasting around 90 seconds. Difficulty talking during contractions, along with the chills or shakes.	In the early phase, try to relax in the comfort of your home and start timing your contractions. Eat something light and stay hydrated. Breathing, relaxation and hydrotherapy techniques may help as the contractions become more intense. Gravity-assisted positions (e.g. squatting or semi-reclined) and walking may be more comfortable. Pain-reducing interventions may be required (or desired).
#2 Pushing & Birth of Your Baby	Baby is moving down the birth canal.	Your baby's head can be felt between your legs and you will have a strong urge to push and/or to have a bowel movement. You may also experience a hot and stinging sensation in your vagina.	Push when instructed to do so (refer to the proper technique described later in the chapter). Gravity-assisted positions can facilitate the baby's descent and can ease the pressure from your pelvis.
#3 Delivery of the Placenta	Uterus continues to contract and the placenta starts to remove itself from the wall of the uterus.	Mild contractions and pushing sensation.	Embrace and bond with your baby. It is the perfect distraction while your doctor does most of the work for you.

*How fast a woman progresses through the stages varies from woman to woman and from pregnancy to pregnancy.

The Link Between Exercise and Labour

There are mixed findings among the numerous studies and reviews on exercise and labour; some studies reported positive relationships, whereas others have found no such relationships. In some of his earlier research, Dr. James Clapp, author of the book *Exercising Through Your Pregnancy*, compared the following 2 groups of women: those who did not exercise during their pregnancy and those who continued to be active throughout their entire pregnancy. His findings were encouraging and showed that active women had an increased incidence (more than 30%) of natural delivery. They also tended to have an easier, shorter and less complicated labour (Table 12.1).

Table 12.1: Summary of Clapp's Findings

Effects of Exercise on the Course of Labour
35% decrease in the need for pain relief
75% decrease in the incidence of maternal exhaustion
50% decrease in the need to artificially rupture the membranes
50% decrease in the need to either induce or stimulate labour with Pitocin
55% decrease in the need for episiotomy
75% decrease in the need for operative interventions (forceps or caesarean section)

Although his results are positive, Clapp cautioned that his studies were limited to a very specific population. For instance, his studies did not look at women that initiated an exercise program once they were pregnant, and therefore, it is unknown whether they would experience the same benefits. It is also interesting to note that previously active women who stopped exercising mid-way through their pregnancy did not experience the benefits described above.

> **Fit for Labour**
> My labour with my first child lasted 30 hours, including 4 hours of pushing. The doctor said that this was some type of record and that the only reason I was able to stay strong enough for this (and avoid a caesarean) was because of my fitness.
> *Andrea M., Ironman triathlete and mother of 2*

More recently, Domenjoz et al. (2014) did a review of the available literature to evaluate the effects of structured exercise programs during pregnancy on the course of labour and delivery. Although they found similar findings with respect to a lower risk of caesarean delivery for women who exercise, the authors found that there was insufficient data to draw conclusions on the rate of episiotomy or epidurals, as well as the length and induction of labour. Once again, we are left with multiple studies showing differing results. Rather than focusing on the differences, take notice of the following take-away-messages:

- Many of the studies show *positive* associations. Generally, staying active throughout your pregnancy seems to lead to certain benefits for your labour.
- Although some studies found no such associations to support the reported benefits, *no studies found that exercise during pregnancy had a negative impact on labour and delivery.*

All the more reason to stay active during your pregnancy!

What's Considered Full Term?

Previously, babies born anywhere between weeks 37-42 was considered "term". But that may now be outdated wisdom. As published in the *Journal Obstetrics & Gynecology* in 2013 and endorsed by ACOG and the Society for Maternal-Fetal Medicine, the definition of term has been updated and it now includes early term, full term, late term and post term.

- Early term – beginning of 37 until the end of 38 weeks gestation
- Full term – beginning of 39 until the end of 40 weeks gestation
- Late term – beginning of 41 weeks until the end of 41 weeks gestation
- Post term – beginning of 42 weeks and beyond

So, when is the most ideal time to give birth? Although you can give birth to a healthy baby anywhere from 37-42 weeks gestation, recent studies have shown that babies born at the beginning of 39 weeks until the end of 40 weeks (full term) have fewer health complications, such as respiratory distress.

Leveraging Your Racing Tactics

Bringing a child into the world is one of life's most amazing miracles. However, many women admit to feeling scared, nervous or anxious about their upcoming labour and delivery. Such feelings are normal and to be expected, given that there are many questions and uncertainties (not to mention pain) with childbirth. One such uncertainty is not knowing *exactly* when the baby will arrive. According to midwife Natalie Wright, a woman has a 94% chance of going into labour between the

37th and 42nd week. This "window of unknown" can be challenging for some women and, in her experience, more so with athletes. "Athletes, in general, are accustomed to setting up a training schedule based on a very specific due date (i.e. the day of their race). Athletes know what they need to do to prepare and can work backwards from the specific day of their race," explains Wright. "This gives them a sense of control. With labour, there is no firm due date; the baby could arrive anywhere in that 4-5 week window."

Fortunately, your athletic experience with training and racing can come in handy and may alleviate some of the fear, nervousness and anxiety, as there are certain similarities between giving birth and performing a challenging workout or race. For instance, both events require planning and patience. Just as you may have spent weeks or months preparing for an upcoming race, you are now spending up to 9 months getting ready for the "big push". Furthermore, despite all your preparations leading up to the event, what actually happens on that particular day is dictated by factors that are both within and beyond your control. During a running race, for instance, you have control over the pace that you will be running and how much fluid you will be consuming. However, you have no control over the weather conditions on that particular day, which, as we know, can have significant consequences for your performance. Similarly, you may have decided that you want a vaginal birth but an emergency caesarean may be required if your baby's heart rate suddenly drops significantly, indicating fetal distress.

You can "borrow" some of the strategies that you use when preparing for an upcoming race and apply them toward your impending labour and delivery. Here's how:

- *Prepare yourself in advance.* Understand the different phases of labour, including what to expect and when (Table 12.0). Consider taking a tour of the hospital or birthing centre where you will be giving birth. Just as it is helpful to know the route and details of the race ahead of time, it can be comforting to be familiar with the surroundings and the general stages of childbirth. Finally, it can be helpful to educate yourself about various activities and strategies that can potentially make your labour easier. Some examples include staying active, strengthening your pelvic floor muscles, stretching your perineum muscles (to reduce the risk of tearing or trauma to the area) and learning about preferred birthing positions. Speak to your doctor or midwife to learn more.

- *Identify your game plan.* As an athlete, you probably found it helpful (and reassuring) to have some sort of plan that outlined how you were going to approach your race. For instance, what pace would you be starting off with and when would you start to go faster? How much fluid should you drink and when? Identifying such strategies ahead of time helps to diminish any anxieties, making you feel more in control of your race. The same concept applies to giving birth; a birthing plan can provide a similar reassurance by outlining your preferences regarding your labour and delivery. Do you want a natural birth? What are your feelings toward medical interventions and pain medication? Who do you want present? A birthing plan can also help to manage realistic expectations - especially as it relates to dealing with the unexpected during labour. Midwife Julie Toole recalls working with 3 elite athletes one summer who were each surprised (and disappointed) with how tough giving birth was and their lack of control on the progression of their labour. Her clients expected labour to be much easier, given their prior training and racing experience. "There are many wild cards in childbirth," explains Toole. "It is important to be prepared to deal with the unexpected and reconcile that there may be changes of plan. Developing a birthing plan and prioritizing certain aspects of it (an A, B, and C goal) and reviewing it with your partner and care provider can help with just that."

My Story: Hill Repeats and Contractions?
As crazy as it sounds, I drew upon my experience as a runner and visualized running hill repeats for each of my contractions. Similar to running up a hard, steep hill, I knew that it was easier to take it 1 hill, or in this case, 1 contraction at a time and to simply focus on getting to the top of the hill or to the end of the contraction. After that, I welcomed a little break before it was time to start the next one. This visualization gave me the confidence that I could get through childbirth...1 contraction at a time.
Jennifer Faraone, co-author, competitive duathlete and runner, mother of 2

- ***Chant your mantras.*** Do you have certain key words or phrases that you say to yourself during a race or a challenging workout to keep you strong and motivated? Statements such as *"I am strong"*, *"Bring it on"* or *"Persevere"* can help to ward off negative thoughts and provide an added boost when things become challenging. This is a common and effective strategy used among many athletes and can also be quite useful during your labour. The trick is to figure out ahead of time which phrases will keep you strong and focused during the most challenging and tiring aspects of labour and delivery. Include your mantras in your birthing plan and share them with your partner, as he or she can then say them with you (or *to you* if you are too tired to say them).

- ***Eat well and stay hydrated.*** Just as you would not want to start a race dehydrated or in a calorie-depleted state, the same concept applies to the days leading up to and during childbirth. When you know that your labour is imminent, make sure that you are well hydrated and that you are continuing to eat healthy. Keeping your energy stores high will help to provide strength and stamina, especially if you experience a very long labour. Keep in mind that you may not feel like eating as your labour progresses and the contractions intensify, so try to eat more in the earlier phases. Foods that you are already familiar with and tend to be easier to digest, such as crackers or a banana, are good first choices. However, you may find that you are craving something entirely different. In her experience as a doula, Adrienne McRuvie has found that most women would rather consume fluids or any type of food that helps to moisten their mouth, such as ice chips or frozen pieces of fruit, especially as their labour progresses. Sipping fluids, ideally something with simple carbohydrates and small amount of sodium, every 10-20 minutes will help avoid dehydration, feeling weak or fevered. Simply wetting your palate helps to moisten your dry mouth, thereby making it easier to breathe and feel more refreshed and energized, explains McRuvie. Although the restriction of fluids and food during labour has traditionally been a common practice across many birth settings, new evidence, including a recent systematic review in the Cochrane Collaboration involving 3130 women in active labour, shows that there is no justification for this restriction in women who are at low risk for complications during delivery. In her experience as a midwife, Wright has found that not eating or drinking can actually impede the progress of labour and potentially increase the need for intervention. But there are some circumstances, including a planned caesarean, where your health care provider may want you on a specific diet; in such cases, it is important to speak to them beforehand.

- **Rest up.** Just like racing, labour and delivery is a mentally and physically exhausting event. In the days and weeks prior to a race or competition, you will have made a conscious effort to start preparing (or tapering) for the event by getting a proper night's sleep, sneaking in some extra rest breaks throughout the day and decreasing the quantity/intensity of your workouts. Similarly, it is important to ensure you get proper rest and potentially modify your activities in the weeks leading up to your targeted delivery date. "I intentionally decreased the intensity and duration of my activity as I approached my delivery date to ensure that I would have enough in the tank for labour," explains Krista Duchene, one of Canada's top marathoners and mother of 3.

> **What Our Athletic Moms Say**
> Here's what some athletes said about their experience with training and childbirth:
>
> - There's no doubt in my mind that my ability to push through intense workouts and competitions gave me the mental and physical toughness needed to tolerate a natural birth. *Stephanie Hewitt, world champion squash player, mother of 3*
> - In my case, no amount of training or activity helped with my labour! Giving birth 3 times was the most tremendous amount of pain I'd ever experienced. No marathon could even compare with it. *Krista DuChene, professional marathoner, mother of 3*
> - I am not sure I would have ever been able to handle labour if I had not been used to the tremendous pain threshold I built up over the years. I knew it had to be over at some point and I just stayed focused on getting there. *Amy Lyman Nedeau, competitive swimmer, mother of 1*
> - As athletes, we are used to pushing through the pain because we know the finish line is near. Giving birth is a similar experience. *Christine Wallace, triathlete and runner, mother of 1*

- *Visualize.* Visualizing before an upcoming race can be an effective way to build your confidence and calm any pre-race jitters. This technique can also be applied to childbirth by mentally walking through the event in a calm and reassuring manner. To practice, simply find a quiet spot, close your eyes and imagine being in labour. Think about what your body will feel like and the strategies that you will use, including mantras, breathing techniques and the different positions you want to incorporate. Imagine yourself strong and in control of the situation, taking one contraction at a time. Finally, visualize the best part - the beautiful baby you will meet for the first time!

- *Believe in yourself!* Above all else, trust and have faith in yourself that you CAN handle this. You have pushed through some hard workouts in the past and have dug deep within yourself to get across the finish line. When it comes time for delivery, have confidence that your body and mind will know what is required to produce a strong finish.

Moan Don't Scream

If you think back to most Hollywood movies involving a woman in labour, more often than not there is a lot of screaming going on in the delivery room. In real life, however, screaming may not be the best choice. Rather, moaning is a technique often promoted in labour, more so by midwives and doulas. Why?

According to Wright, moaning has a more relaxing and opening effect on the body, in comparison to screaming. Think about it: screaming is a fight or flight reactionary response that is characterized by a high-pitched tone that comes from a place of anxiety and fear. When you scream, you create tension in your body, which is the opposite of how you want your body to respond during labour. But moaning, on the other hand, is characterized by low-pitched tones and is a more controlled and intentional reaction, promoting a greater sense of calm and safety. Wright further explains that moaning can trigger a natural instinct to crouch down and squat, which can also be helpful during labour.

McRuvie also encourages women to moan during labour. McRuvie explains that there is a natural connection between the face and the rest of the body. "As you relax your face, such as with a moan, your body naturally follows suit - including your pelvic floor muscles. The opposite happens when you scream; your face tenses and the rest of your body tightens," explains McRuvie. Jaclyn Kissel, a former sprinter who currently trains for triathlons and mother of 1, followed this advice during her recent labour. "The notion of moaning, rather than screaming, really made sense to me; I lost my voice from moaning by the end, but it worked!"

Training Your Muscles to Push Properly
In the chapter "Your Strong And Powerful Core" we used the analogy of squeezing toothpaste out of its tube to explain the importance of your abdominal and pelvic floor muscles working *together* to help with the pushing phase of childbirth. Your abdominal muscles will need to contract to help push the baby out, while at the same time your pelvic floor muscles will need to relax so that the baby can pass through the vaginal canal more easily. Otherwise, tight pelvic floor muscles may make childbirth more difficult. It is in your best interest to learn how to work both muscles groups together.

In theory this might seem easy but, in fact, it can be a bit hard to execute. Let us demonstrate: as you are sitting here reading this book, slowly exhale and pull your belly button into your spine (such as when you are anticipating a punch to the stomach) and hold. Now, contract your pelvic floor muscles (imagine "pulling them up"). Finally, without releasing your abdominal muscles, relax the pelvic floor muscles. How did you find this? If you are like most women, it may have been a bit challenging. But relax –practice makes perfect! This is where the Birth Preparation Routine comes into play (Appendix 6), as it outlines a series of exercises that will help you activate and coordinate your abdominal and pelvic floor muscles to facilitate childbirth. Remember that this coordination between your abdominal and pelvic floor muscles will not necessarily happen on its own. Similar to any other muscle that you expect to perform, you will need to train these muscles first before expecting them to help you in the delivery room. It is strongly recommended that you first read the chapter "Your Silent Training Partner - Your Pelvic Floor Muscles" to review how to perform the pelvic floor strengthening exercises correctly.

Summary
After 9 months of anticipation, the big day will finally arrive. Fortunately, your experience and fitness as an athlete can work in your favour. If you

were able to remain active throughout your entire pregnancy, you may be more likely to experience some potential benefits such as a decreased chance of complications and medical interventions. Since no studies have found that exercising will hinder your labour and delivery, this is all the more reason to stay active during your pregnancy - in case you were not convinced already! Furthermore, the tactics that you apply in preparation for an upcoming sporting event, like visualization, repeating key phrases, and creating an execution plan can come in handy as you prepare for the biggest event of your life. Finally, don't forget about the Birth Preparation Routine found in Appendix 6 – practice really does make perfect!

GETTING YOUR GROOVE BACK

Chapter 13

A HOLISTIC APPROACH TO GETTING YOUR GROOVE BACK

When can I start exercising again?
Why can't I simply just pick up from where I left off?
What factors do I need to consider when getting back into training?

It May Not Be as Simple as You Think
The questions above may reflect what you, and other athletic moms, ask within the days, weeks and months after giving birth. It is actually not uncommon to have a desire to participate in some form of light exercise (as opposed to a structured and strenuous training program) at this time. Whether it stems from the need to have some well-deserved "me" time, an outlet to cope with all the changes, a desire to feel good about your body or a way to regain a sense of control, you may crave, want and *need* to exercise. Such a desire is a good thing, as there are many benefits to exercising postpartum, including:

- Decreasing your chances for postpartum depression.
- Increasing your energy levels and your overall mood.
- Improving overall body strength and posture.
- Regaining your pre-pregnancy body faster.
- Promoting a faster recovery.
- Helping to prevent the onset of, or lessen the symptoms associated with common postpartum conditions such as low back pain, headaches, incontinence, varicose veins, leg pain and painful intercourse.

However, starting to exercise postpartum is not simply a matter of putting on your exercise gear and heading out to the local gym, pool or track. Although this may be the approach that some women take, you will soon learn why this may not be a good idea - especially if you want to avoid setbacks, injuries, frustration and disappointment.

> **The Difference Between Training and Exercising**
> We differentiate between the terms exercising and training. *Training* is characterized by your commitment to some form of a plan that enables you to work toward a specific goal and may include larger volume and/or more intense activity. *Exercising* is used to describe your intention to incorporate physical activity in a less-scheduled manner, without a concrete goal or expectation.

Looking for Guidance

Many women simply jump back into an exercise routine as soon as they feel that the timing is right. This is not surprising, given that there is little information available on postpartum exercise. In fact, most guidelines on postpartum exercise are less descriptive than those for pregnancy, and the majority of resources including books, articles, websites and research studies rarely expand beyond the following:

- Wait until you have received medical clearance from your doctor before starting an exercise program.
- Start off easy and gradually increase the duration, frequency and intensity, as tolerated.
- Avoid exercising if you experience pain or heavy bleeding.
- Ensure adequate food and fluid intake.
- Get plenty of rest.
- Avoid doing anything that does not feel right.

> **Letting the Body Heal**
> Looking back, I realize that I probably exercised more than what my body was ready for, as my bleeding would increase significantly after working out. It was not about trying to lose the weight or regaining my fitness as fast as possible; rather, I jumped back into training so soon because I missed that comforting and familiar feeling of working out and doing something that was purely for me. I have since realized the importance of respecting my body more and giving it the proper time to heal.
> *Seanna Keating, elite squash player and mother of 3*

Although such advice is accurate and may be adequate for many women, the information is somewhat vague, providing very little guidance in terms of the quantity and intensity of exercise. It also does not take into consideration the different types of exercise, such as low versus high impact sports or activities. For instance, your body might be able to handle a more intense swim workout 4 weeks postpartum but it may need more time to withstand the stress and impact of a hard running workout. In addition, the general recommendations listed above do not take into account non-physical factors, like your level of motivation and personal circumstances that can influence your desire and ability to resume exercising and training. Finally, some athletes, especially professional or sponsored ones, may feel they are expected to return to their training as soon as possible. For instance, Karen Cockburn, trampolinist, Olympic medalist and mother of 1, had to reach a certain fitness level 9 months postpartum in order to keep her status as a carded athlete with Sports Canada.

So what is the best way to start exercising again and take your fitness to a level that provides you with personal satisfaction? How do you ensure that this is done in a safe manner without putting you at risk of injury? More importantly, how do you balance the demands of both motherhood and training?

Everyone Is Different

Scenario 1: Jane is feeling great, both emotionally and physically, and has started training again with a personal trainer.

Scenario 2: Mary Anne's baby is crying all the time. She is exhausted and although she really misses the training, she does not have the energy to exercise.

Scenario 3: Susan has tried, on several occasions, to go jogging but found it uncomfortable and even painful at times.

These scenarios illustrate that every woman has a different postpartum experience. This is one of the reasons why it can be challenging to provide detailed guidelines for postpartum exercise. Rather than comparing yourself to others, realize that you are a unique individual and applaud the small improvements that you make every day.

A More Holistic and Gradual Approach

Resuming an exercise or training program is not just a matter of waiting until you feel physically ready; using this marker alone can be misleading. You should not assume that your body's ability to tolerate day-to-day activities, such as grocery shopping and playing with your child, is a sign that your body can handle the physical demands of exercise. Furthermore, physical readiness is different from emotional readiness. Although your body may be physically ready, you may not be motivated to start exercising, let alone training, in a consistent manner. Your reasons for wanting to start exercising again may be driven by motivations that are less than ideal. Are you preoccupied with losing the baby weight as fast as possible? Are you feeling pressured by your sponsors, coaches or teammates to start training as soon as possible? Such reasons put you at risk of doing too much, too soon, resulting in injury. Ultimately, you may lose the enjoyment that you once cherished participating in your training.

Finally, there is an additional factor to consider - your situational readiness. This simply means that although you may be physically and emotionally ready to start training again, there are other factors that will either facilitate or hinder your ability to train. These could include limited childcare and supportive networks, disrupted sleep or breastfeeding schedules. Many moms will agree that balancing both motherhood and training can be challenging. Although there are multiple ways to set up an exercise or training program, the key is finding the setup that works best for you and your family. Such a set up may be very different from what you were accustomed to prior to starting a family. "My approach to training has definitely changed since having kids, and more so now that I am back at work. There are days when I would just rather hang out with my children than head out to train," explains Wendy Simms, 5-time Canadian national cyclocross champion and mother of 2. "I now use local events to "race into shape". They are fun, I get in a great workout, I'm surrounded by others with a similar passion and I'm setting a good example for my kids."

Figuring out the right set up for your training may take a bit of time and patience. So remember, when

> ### No Easy Feat
> No one ever said that balancing training and motherhood would be easy! In fact, the most challenging time to stay committed to an exercise or training program is probably during the postpartum period, given your new time constraints and demands of motherhood. In a survey conducted in 2005 that examined physical activity levels in the postpartum period, researchers found that almost 2/3 of new moms identified themselves as "inactive" after childbirth. Furthermore, close to ½ of women that were fit prior to pregnancy classified themselves as "inactive" or "irregularly active" after giving birth. The main reasons for this lack of physical activity were personal issues, insufficient support from their spouses and their new parenting responsibilities.

deciding when and how to start exercising and training, it is helpful to consider:

- *Your physical readiness* to handle the day-to-day activities and the physical demands of exercising.
- *Your emotional readiness* including your desire and motivation to exercise and train again.
- *Your situational readiness* or your personal circumstances that can either hinder or facilitate your return to training.

We therefore recommend that you apply a gradual, rather than an all-or-nothing, approach to regaining your fitness and performance levels. We encourage you to look at your training as a series of building blocks that begins the moment you give birth and helps you progress over the coming weeks and months (Figure 13.0).

PHASE 1:

YOUR INITIAL RECOVERY
- Immediately after birth; focus is on you and your baby.
- Purpose of **activity** is to promote healing and regain strength for your role as a mom.

PHASE 2:

YOUR ONGOING RECOVERY & LIGHT EXERCISE
- You are still recovering yet feeling stronger and in more control.
- Purpose of **exercise** is to build fitness and establish light exercise routine that satisfies you.

PHASE 3:

YOUR STRUCTURED TRAINING PROGRAM
- You are feeling emotionally and physically strong.
- Purpose of structured and more intense **training** is to work toward achieving your specific goals while balancing the needs of your family.

Figure 13.0: 3 Phases To Your Postpartum Comeback

We have intentionally made little reference to "time" when defining these 3 phases, as there is so much variability that exists from one woman to another and even from one pregnancy to another. Rather, each phase has been described with its own purpose and characteristics that, in turn, should help you determine the appropriate timing of initiating and increasing your activity levels.

Sounds like a lot of information to digest? You bet! This is why "getting your groove back" may be more complicated than you thought. We hope to make this easier by breaking up the information into manageable sections:

- A chapter providing an overview of the primary changes and transformations that your body experiences within the weeks and months following childbirth.
- Three separate chapters detailing the descriptions of the 3 phases to getting your groove back.
- A chapter offering important information and helpful strategies about ways to enhance the breastfeeding experience while resuming your training.

So make yourself comfortable - and start reading!

What Worked for Me

Danelle Kabush never doubted that she would return to some level of training after her pregnancy. However, she was not sure if, and when, she would be motivated to resume competing. This changed when she was offered a contract with the Luna Pro Team a month after giving birth and was soon back in racing shape. "I viewed the sponsorship with Luna as an amazing opportunity to resume training and competing as quickly as I could but within reason. I follow the philosophy that if I stop being motivated, if I'm not having fun competing, and if it is not working for my family, then it is time to stop," she explains. Although Kabush's story may not apply to all women, it speaks to the idea that getting back into training and racing postpartum is not just a matter of physical readiness, it is also about motivation and finding out what works for you and your family.

Danelle Kabush, professional XTERRA triathlete and mother of 2

Chapter 14

RESPECTING YOUR NEW BODY

How long will it take for my body to return to "normal"?
How will this impact my ability to train again?
What are the risks with starting too soon?

Managing Realistic Expectations

We deliberately chose "respecting" for the title of this chapter to emphasize your body's ongoing transformation following childbirth and we encourage you to treat it accordingly. Let's face it: many athletes, yourself included, may have high expectations when it comes to their body's ability to recuperate from physically challenging workouts. How many times have you pushed your body through a challenging workout, only to repeat a similar workout after a day or two of rest? However, your body's ability to quickly bounce back after an intense workout does not necessarily mean that you can expect that same pattern following childbirth. In fact, you may be surprised with the amount of time your body now needs to recuperate properly. Deborah Moore, an Ironman athlete, coach and mother of 3, was surprised with how exhausted she was within the first week of giving birth. "Given my past experience as an athlete, I thought that I would have been able to handle a short walk around the block. I was wrong and had to take a break after 3 minutes".

Managing realistic expectations may also be influenced by the media. Consider for a moment the media frenzy surrounding famous actresses who have lost their baby weight in record time. Or the attention some professional athletes receive after winning a major event within the first year of having a baby. Paula Radcliffe, a British marathoner, received international attention after winning the New York City marathon just 10 months after giving birth to her first child. Rather than comparing yourself to such individuals, keep in mind that "their body" is their job and that they have an army of people (e.g. personal chefs, trainers and nannies) to help them achieve their fitness goals and to look "*good*" in the public eye. Instead, celebrate the person you are, knowing that your temporary weight gain was for a very good cause and your future athletic accomplishments are just around the corner.

Finally, any high expectations that you have of your body's ability to recuperate quickly may stem from your high level of motivation. After many months of reduced (or very little) activity, you might be ready to start again. It can be easy to let this enthusiasm drive your decision toward when and how to start your training. Remember that your body took 9 months to undergo this wonderful transformation and then went through a physically challenging (and perhaps traumatic) labour. Time and patience are a must. Remember that each person is different and that your weight loss and postpartum fitness will return in due course.

> **Had I Been More Patient**
> I may have pushed my running a bit too soon after my pregnancy. My goal was to run a qualifying marathon for the London Olympics 9 months after giving birth to my son. This was perhaps too much pressure on my body and I ended up with sacroiliac (pelvic) joint problems. Unfortunately, I had to pull out of the race and missed the next 2 months of training.
> *Mary Davies, elite marathoner and soon-to-be mother of 2*

Understanding Your Transforming Body

Just as you learned earlier about your body's transformation during pregnancy, it is important to have a similar understanding of what is happening to your body within the days, weeks and even months following childbirth. Dr. Julia Alleyne, a sport and exercise physician who has worked with several Olympic athletes throughout their pregnancies and postpartum periods, explains that pregnancy should be viewed beyond the traditional 9-month duration, as the body continues to transform for quite some time following childbirth. The timing of such a transformation can be influenced by a variety of things including hormonal and lifestyle factors that many new mothers face, such as disrupted sleep and mental exhaustion. As such, Alleyne suggests that women consider pregnancy to be 12-24 months in duration. Furthermore, it is also important to realize that your body may never be the same as it was prior to pregnancy and you may have to understand what your "new normal" will be.

The following list describes the more common changes that your body may be experiencing now and in the coming months. Rather than including all of the possible changes, we have focused on those that could have the greatest implications for your daily activities and training ambitions.

Vaginal Bleeding
It is normal to continue bleeding in the days and weeks after giving birth. This discharge, known as lochia, is a combination of blood and the remainder of the uterine lining from your pregnancy. The heavy bleeding normally stops after 2-4 weeks. However, it can come and go for a few months. You should contact your doctor immediately if you experience heavy bleeding (e.g. soaking a pad in 15 minutes), as it might indicate ripped stitches or a blood clot. If your bleeding increases during or after your exercise, it is most likely a sign that your body is not yet ready for this type or intensity of exercise. If you experience increased bleeding, stop exercising and rest for a few days before trying the activity again. You may also need to start exercising at a lesser intensity and build up gradually.

Loosened Ligaments and Joints
It is unknown how long relaxin remains elevated in your body following childbirth. Reports suggest that this hormone, which was responsible for relaxing your pelvic and other joints in preparation for childbirth, can remain in the body up to a year following delivery. The point to remember is that your joints may still be lax (or loose) for several months after the birth of your child, possibly affecting your ability to perform activities (exercise, sports, day-to-day activities) and increasing your risk of injury. Not stretching past the point of resistance, avoiding any jerky movements or sudden changes in direction, and being extra cautious when on uneven terrain can help to minimize your risk of injury.

Breast Soreness and Engorgement
Your milk supply starts to come in within the first 24-72 hours after giving birth, making your breast quite swollen, engorged and tender.

Breastfeeding may leave your nipples dry, cracked and sore. All of this can be a source of discomfort and can limit the timing of your daily activities, not to mention your workouts. Placing ice packs on your breasts following breastfeeding can help to reduce swelling, whereas taking a hot shower or using warm compresses prior to breastfeeding may help your milk flow. Regular use of a topical breast cream to relieve dry, cracked nipples, wearing a sport bra with added support when exercising and scheduling your workouts after a feeding are other helpful strategies. See your doctor if you suspect that you have mastitis, an infection of the breast tissue that results in breast pain, swelling, warmth, redness, hardness and possibly, a fever.

Upper Back Aches and Pains

You likely spend a lot of time bending over your child – feeding, changing diapers, bathing etc. Not surprisingly, you may have noticed new aches and pains, especially in your midback or between your shoulder blades. Such aches and pains relate to the increased amount of time that you spend in a hunched or bent over position, causing your pectoralis (or chest) muscles to tighten and causing the opposing muscles, your lower trapezius and rhomboid (or midback) muscles to weaken. Over time, these muscular changes may cause poor posture or postural imbalance, thereby causing pain. The good news is there are a few simple exercises you can do to help alleviate these new pains; refer to Appendix 7 "Stop Breaking Your (Upper) Back, Baby".

Internal Organs and Surrounding Connective Tissues

As your baby was growing inside your belly, some of your internal organs, such as your intestines, stomach and diaphragm, shifted positions and/or moved upward. These organs then start to settle back to their normal position following childbirth. How long it takes for things to settle depends on a variety of factors and is very individualized, explains Pam Ennis, an osteopath who has worked with numerous pregnant and athletic women. Ennis cautions that this shifting may cause a temporary misalignment or unnecessary tension in your body, potentially leading to muscle imbalances and injuries. This makes it increasingly important to avoid the temptation of rushing back to your sport or exercise regime too quickly and to give your body the time it needs to find its "new normal", especially in the lower back and abdominal areas.

Body Weight Changes

There are no hard and fast rules when it comes to how long it takes to lose the baby weight. Dr. James Clapp, author of Exer*cising Through Your Pregnancy*, estimates that it can take, on average, 6-12 months to resume your pre-pregnancy body weight and to restore the tone in your abdomen. Furthermore, there are a number of factors, including your activity levels, calorie intake, hormonal fluctuations and breastfeeding that may affect your weight. Focusing on your pre-pregnancy weight may not be suitable at this time; a more appropriate goal might be to ensure healthy eating habits and moderate activity or exercise, while trusting that the appropriate weight loss will follow.

Knee Pain

Mild to moderate knee pain can be common if you are still carrying some extra weight and if your ligaments are still lax due to the hormone relaxin. Such pain may be greater with weight-bearing activities and high-impact sports such as running. Strengthening the muscles around the knees and wearing shoes with proper support may help to alleviate this issue.

Reduced Abdominal Strength and Tone

It has been weeks or months since you have given birth, so why does it still look like you are several months pregnant, despite your efforts to eat a proper diet and adopt a core strengthening routine? Seana Zelazo, Olympic trial marathoner runner and mother of 1, thought her stomach would get back to its pre-pregnancy state much faster. "I was expecting my stomach to be flatter by the time my son was 3 months old. Most of my pregnancy weight was in my stomach, so toning the abdominal muscles and losing the last 5 lbs. was my main focus," explains Zelazo.

> **It Took a While**
>
> Following the birth of her 1st child, Canadian Olympic hurdler Priscilla Lopes-Schliep was back to training within 4 weeks to prepare for the upcoming 2012 Olympics. Although she was pleased with her overall training and progress, she was a bit surprised with the additional time it took for her abdominal muscles to restore their tone. "I felt uncomfortable posing for pictures at first, since my abs were not what they used to be. I learned to accept that the tone would come back in due course."
> *Priscilla Lopes-Schliep, Olympic hurdler and mother of 2*

Such expectations are common, even though they may not be realistic for most people. Think of your pregnant stomach as a balloon that slowly inflates as your baby grows. During childbirth, your balloon did not suddenly "pop". Rather, it started a slow leak, leaving with you a stomach that is quite soft, squishy and weak. Although losing your belly bulge goes hand in hand with losing weight, part of it has to do with the time it takes for your uterus to gradually shrink back to it is normal size. Your uterus expanded to a size large enough to hold 2 large bottles of pop! It then takes 4-6 weeks for your uterus to shrink from 2-2.5 lbs. to 0.5 lbs. or less.

A condition called diastasis recti (the separation of the rectus abdominis muscle) also affects the firmness and strength of your abdominal muscles. Studies suggest that 53% of women may experience this condition in the postpartum period. Women with this condition often complain of their inability to tone their abdominal muscles, despite their best efforts. Not only does this affect the way that your stomach looks, more importantly diastasis recti weakens your entire core strength and can lead to a series of problems, including low back pain. For some women, diastasis recti may resolve naturally anywhere from 1 day to 8 weeks following birth. However, those who do not see improvement may require the help of a qualified professional. More information about this condition can be found in the chapter "Your Strong And Powerful Core".

Back Pain and Pelvic Girdle Pain
As discussed in the chapter "Getting Sidelined", low back pain (LBP) and pelvic girdle pain (PGP) are very common during pregnancy. Now that you have given birth, these issues may still occur. However, as a new mother, you may be more likely to experience LBP than PGP, as this condition can affect up to 25% of women in the postpartum period. It has been suggested that these conditions are a result of your abdominal muscles being stretched over the course of your pregnancy, along with the added workload of your back muscles to maintain proper posture. As a result, you may feel extra pain in your lower back and pelvic area.

Although it is important to give your body time to recuperate from pregnancy and childbirth and regain its strength, it is equally important to maintain proper posture throughout your daily activities (e.g. bending over to pick up your newborn child and carrying the car seat). Most aches and pains that you may feel should be temporary and will likely resolve on their own. However, you may find it helpful to seek help from qualified health care professionals such as physiotherapists or chiropractors should the symptoms persist or if they interfere with your daily activities.

Perineum and Pelvic Floor Muscles

Your perineum is the area between your vagina and rectum and it has been through a lot during pregnancy and labour. The muscles may have become weaker as a result of the constant pressure of the uterus and they may have been stretched, traumatized or even torn or cut during labour. Any swelling usually resolves within the first 2 weeks following delivery and most of the muscle tone is regained by 6 weeks, with more improvement over the following months. During this time, it is not uncommon to experience a weak bladder resulting in a loss of urine or the sudden urge to urinate (also known as incontinence). Such symptoms can be set off by sneezing, laughing, jumping and running. Fortunately, many studies suggest that strengthening the pelvic floor muscles within 6 months postpartum significantly improves continence status. In severe cases, or when left unaddressed (e.g. not doing any pelvic floor strengthening exercises), weak pelvic floor muscles can also lead to a prolapsed organ, such as the uterus or bladder. Refer to the chapter "Your Silent Training Partner – Your Pelvic Floor Muscles" to learn more.

It Can Happen to You

Think that a leaky bladder, incontinence or a prolapsed organ only happens to older women? Think again! Unfortunately, pregnancy and vaginal delivery are known risk factors in the development of urinary incontinence. Consider the following information about pregnancy, labour and your pelvic floor muscles:

- The rate of pregnancy and postpartum incontinence is twice that of someone who has not had a child.
- For most women, incontinence resolves within 3 months after delivery, yet it can last up to a year.
- About 10-20% percent of women with a vaginal delivery will be bothered by prolapse by the time they reach the age of 50.

Incontinence, prolapse and the feeling that "things just aren't right down there" can be unpleasant, discouraging and inconvenient. The good news is that in many cases, such conditions or symptoms are temporary and/or can improve over time. Refer to our chapter "Your Silent Training Partner - Your Pelvic Floor Muscles" for more information.

Hemorrhoids

Hemorrhoids are swollen veins in the rectum and can be common as a result of pushing during labour or from the constipation that you may experience during pregnancy and/or following childbirth. High impact sports, such as running on hard surfaces or prolonged sitting on a narrow seat like a bike seat, may further worsen the symptoms. Although hemorrhoids can be permanent, wearing clothing that will not irritate the area (such as loose fitting underwear), running on softer surfaces and using a padded bike seat may help to lessen or alleviate the symptoms. Taking a sitz bath (or sitting in water up to the hips) can help keep the area clean and promote blood circulation. Eating fibre-rich foods and drinking lots of water can help to minimize straining during bowel movements. Finally, an over-the-counter stool softener may be helpful should the above not work.

It's Worth the Wait

As discussed above, your body is a wonderful mechanism that can handle a tremendous amount of change. What's even more amazing is that your body does a terrific job of letting these changes settle and promoting its own healing as it finds its "new normal". The key to this healing, however, is *time*. You simply cannot force your body to heal faster than it can handle. Radcliffe, the elite runner we referred to at the beginning of the chapter, had an amazing race performance shortly after giving birth. However, this did not come without a price - including a stress fracture in her pelvis shortly afterward. She believes this injury was a result of doing too much too soon, as revealed by Radcliffe in an interview with the Guardian Newspaper in 2010. However, it is not just your body that you need to be paying attention to. It is all too easy to let your mind dictate the timing of your return to exercise, which can be influenced by external pressures such as sponsors, as well as your own personal ambitions. Time and patience are a must, as is really listening to your body. In the end, you will increase your chances of coming back stronger and injury-free.

Knowing if and when your body is ready to handle the physical stress of training can be tricky. Fortunately, there are some general principles and simple checks that may make this transition easier. You may also benefit from the assistance of certain health care professionals, such as chiropractors, physiotherapists and osteopaths, who can ensure your body is on the right track in finding its "new normal". Such considerations, as well as other helpful tips, will be detailed in the following chapters.

Summary

Being aware of the temporary (and sometimes lasting) effects of pregnancy on your body is important. You will be doing yourself a huge favour by respecting what your body has gone through, giving it the time to heal properly and perhaps, seeking help from a qualified health care professional before starting to exercise and resume training. Overall, such patience can go long way in preventing injuries and setbacks, not the mention frustration, now and over the next few months.

Chapter 15

PHASE 1: YOUR INITIAL RECOVERY

Shouldn't all of my attention be on my baby right now?
If I am more fit than the average woman, why can't I start exercising right away?
Are there different considerations if I had a caesarean?

A Critical Time

The first few days and weeks after giving birth are challenging times, as there is so much going on, including the pain or discomfort from labour, the disrupted sleep patterns, the roller coaster of emotions and the sudden reality of caring for your newborn 24/7. Exercise is likely the furthest thing from your mind – as it should be, given that your focus is on caring for your newborn and fostering your own healing. What you may not realize, however, is that these first couple of days and weeks following childbirth are a critical time in your journey back to training, as your actions during this time can have an effect on you months later. This is why we have suggested that your postpartum comeback be gradual, incorporating the 3-phase approach we showed earlier in Figure 13.0.

The next couple of months will take you through a gradual progression of physical activity, beginning with some light activity to promote healing in Phase 1, building toward a structured training program in Phase 3 that will help you achieve your performance goals. Failure to take the necessary time to progress through these phases may result in frustration, disappointment, setbacks and injuries. This progression begins with taking care of yourself in Phase 1: Your Initial Recovery.

As illustrated in Figure 15.0, this phase begins shortly after giving birth and focuses on taking the necessary steps to ensure that you are healing properly, bonding with your child and starting to cope with your new role as a mom.

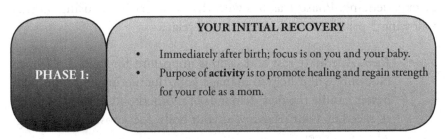

Figure 15.0: Phase 1: Your Initial Recovery

Your Immediate Priorities
There is no doubt that taking care of your little one is now your top priority. However, this does not mean that you should be putting yourself second. In fact, many experts and moms agree that an equally important priority within the first few days and weeks should also include your own recovery. It is common to underestimate the magnitude of the physical and emotional stress of pregnancy and childbirth and assume that you can simply "bounce back" after a few days. Furthermore, it is easy to overlook the fact that what you do in the short-term (i.e. the first couple of days), can have an impact on the long-term (i.e. in the coming months). For instance, not taking the time upfront to rest and ensure adequate sleep may leave you feeling completely exhausted within a couple of weeks. A study published in the New England Journal of

> **When is it Just the Blues?**
> Although you have been blessed with this amazing new bundle of joy, do you sometimes feel depressed, anxious or upset? Relax…this is normal in many instances. Referred to as the "baby blues" or "postpartum blues", many new moms experience a variety of different emotions a few days after giving birth. Some of the common signs include anger, crying for no clear reason, difficulty sleeping, poor appetite, inability to make simple decisions and feelings of doubt about caring for your baby. Such feelings typically come and go over the course of a week or two but usually go away on their own without the need for any treatment. If such feelings worsen or do not go away after a few weeks, please seek help, as it could be a sign of a more serious condition known as postpartum depression.

Medicine found that not allowing time for the body to properly heal might result in a longer recovery period.

It is important to use this time to let your body recover, regain its strength and manage the overwhelming emotions that you may be experiencing. Phase 1 assists with this recovery by focusing on the following 3 priorities: rest, replenish and relate.

- **Rest.** Adequate rest and sleep is important for several reasons. Not only will it help to manage your fluctuating emotions and better handle the new demands of motherhood, it can also help to speed up your recovery, as your body does most of its healing while you sleep.
- **Replenish.** Replenishing yourself with proper food will also support your recovery by making sure that you have the necessary nutrients to promote healing. Furthermore, a proper diet will give you the energy and stamina needed to meet the challenging needs of motherhood and enhance the quality and quantity of your breast milk. Although you might be concerned with losing weight, now is not the time to deprive yourself (or your nursing baby) of much-needed nourishment.
- **Relate.** You have just spent the last 9 months bonding with your child while he/she was in your womb; now, you get to bond with your baby in a completely different way. Relating to and connecting with your child within the first few days is magical and will allow you to get to know this little person.

Reality Check

One of the hardest challenges for some new moms is accepting that they have very little, if any, control of their bodies in the first few days and weeks after giving birth. Deborah Moore, who has completed several Ironmans, was surprised with how exhausted she was within her first few days postpartum. "I thought that my past experience as an athlete, coupled with the fact that I remained active during my pregnancy, would mean that I could handle a short walk the next day with my husband and our new baby girl," explains Moore. "But much to my surprise, I had to take a break after 3 minutes! This is when I realized what a challenge it would be to balance my body's readiness with my mind's readiness."

Deborah Moore, Ironman triathlete, coach and mother of 3

Healing Through Activity

You may have noticed that we use the term "activity" rather than "exercise" in Phase 1. This was a deliberate effort on our part to emphasize the notion that this phase is about moving your body in a gentle and non-stressful manner. The purpose of such activity is not to lose weight or to regain your fitness, but rather to get your blood circulating to promote healing, to begin regaining your strength for everyday activities and to help you function as a new mom. There are a variety of activities that you can do, as long as they are gentle on your body. For instance, the Canadian Society for Exercise Physiology (CSEP) recommends walking, pelvic floor exercises and stretching of all muscle groups. Walking is a great activity at this point as it is convenient, requires no equipment and gives you a chance to leave your house. More importantly, walking is a safe method for assessing your body's status and helps make sure you have not overexerted yourself (Table 15.0). You may be surprised how your body now reacts when trying some form of light activity.

Table 15.0: Signs of Overexertion in the Recovery Phase

One or more of the following signs and symptoms could be an indication that you might have overexerted yourself during light physical activity:

- Increased vaginal bleeding or change in colour (bright red)
- Dizziness
- Faintness
- Joint pain
- Exhaustion
- Increased pelvic pressure

If you experience any of these symptoms during or following your activity, it is important that you stop and rest. Let the symptoms settle for a few days before trying the activity again. Speak to your doctor if the symptoms do not subside.

Giving Some TLC to Your Pelvic Floor Muscles
Although you may be thinking the opposite, now is actually a crucial time to focus on your pelvic floor muscles. These muscles worked hard during the course of your pregnancy and played an important role during labour. By the end of your pregnancy, your pelvic floor muscles are tired, stressed and possibly injured. Like any fatigued or injured muscle, they need time to heal and may require some tender loving care. Initiating light pelvic floor strengthening activities will help to

trigger those muscles again and promote blood circulation, which will further encourage healing in your perineum region. You can start such strengthening activities as early as the next day following childbirth. However, you may be advised to wait and check with your doctor first if you had tearing, extensive stitching or a prolapse.

Dragana Boljanovic-Susic, a physiotherapist who specializes in pelvic floor wellness, encourages new moms to limit prolonged standing or sitting in the first few days following a vaginal delivery. She also suggests resting with your feet elevated and performing pelvic floor strengthening activities several times throughout the day. "Balancing rest and pelvic floor strengthening activities will promote better recovery of your weakened pelvic floor muscles," says Boljanovic-Susic. Working these muscles is also a preventative measure, as it can help to ward off future complications such as urinary incontinence and organ prolapse, which can sometimes occur after pregnancy. A study in the UK found that 87% of women reported some type of perineum problem a year after giving birth; this included women who did not have any tears or an episiotomy during labour.

Hopefully, you were working your pelvic floor muscles on a regular basis during your pregnancy and you are already familiar with such activities (i.e. Kegel exercises). You may find that you are only able to do a few repetitions at first – if so, relax, as that is normal. With a bit of time and effort, you will gradually increase the muscles' endurance and strength. If you have not performed these activities, you can always refer to the chapter "Your Silent Training Partner - Your Pelvic Floor Muscles" for more information.

Additional Considerations With a Caesarean
In comparison to a non-complicated vaginal birth, your recovery time may be longer if you had a caesarean. Surgery places added stress on your abdominal muscles and increases the time needed for your incision to heal. Many doctors suggest waiting 6-8 weeks before starting any form of exercise or waiting until your incision has healed. Consider the following:

- You may be spending additional days in the hospital. Not only are you recovering from childbirth but you are also recovering from major abdominal surgery. Pain management will be important in the first few days after surgery.

- You might be bedridden for days or even weeks and have certain restrictions, such as avoiding heavy household chores or lifting anything heavier than your baby. These restrictions will help to minimize any additional strain on your abdominal muscles.
- Adequate rest becomes even more important, as you will likely feel more tired and your body will need additional time to heal.
- Your abdominal muscles will be very weak following your surgery, thereby offering less support to your lower back. You will need to strengthen your entire core, including your lower back, abdominal and pelvic floor muscles. Refer to the chapter "Your Strong And Powerful Core" for more information.

Summary
Congratulations on becoming a mom! In the first few days and weeks, you will no doubt experience a variety of changes and fluctuating emotions. This critical phase is not just about focusing on your child; it is also about focusing on yourself and ensuring you take the necessary steps to promote healing and begin regaining your strength for everyday activities as a new mom.

Chapter 16

PHASE 2: YOUR ONGOING RECOVERY AND LIGHT EXERCISE

Why is it often recommended to wait 6 weeks before exercising?
What factors influence my readiness?
What can I do to decrease the risk of injuries or setbacks?

Taking It to the Next Level

Have you regained some of your strength and feel relatively rested? Were you able to perform some type of light activity, such as walking, without experiencing any of the signs and symptoms described in Table 15.0? Do you feel like you have regained some control over your life? If so, welcome to Phase 2: Your ongoing recovery & light exercise (Figure 16.0).

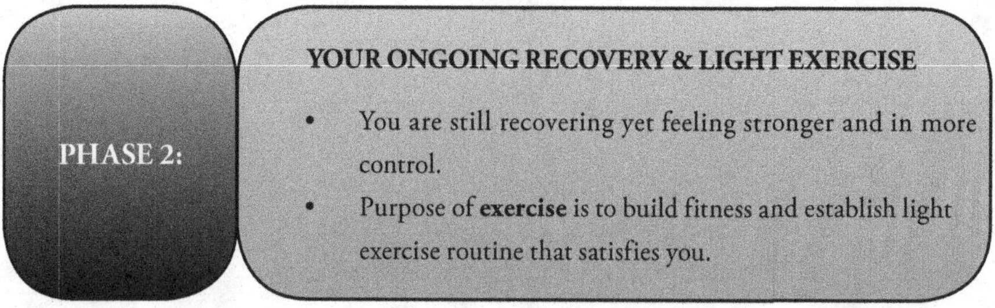

PHASE 2:

YOUR ONGOING RECOVERY & LIGHT EXERCISE

- You are still recovering yet feeling stronger and in more control.
- Purpose of **exercise** is to build fitness and establish light exercise routine that satisfies you.

Figure 16.0: Phase 2: Your Ongoing Recovery & Light Exercise

You are likely ready to engage in some form of *moderate* exercise – including more strenuous forms of weight bearing activities, several times a week. But before jumping out the door to exercise, keep in mind that your body may still be recovering from pregnancy and childbirth. You may also be continuing to settle into a routine as a new mom. Not surprisingly, the risk of emotional and physical burnout at this time is high. As such, the goal of Phase 2 is to establish an exercise routine that promotes moderate fitness and makes you feel good about yourself. It is also about carving out time for yourself on a consistent basis and doing something that you find enjoyable, as opposed to striving for peak fitness. Gradually losing some of the excess weight (if any) may become a secondary goal but should not take priority. Morgan, a competitive swimmer and mother of 2, jumped on the elliptical machine shortly after giving birth. "It was not about losing weight or getting in a tough workout," Morgan explains. "I simply needed to feel like myself and to take back some of the control over my life."

Phase 2 is also an important building block for the 3rd phase - initiating a structured training program - as it provides an opportunity to "test out the water" and see how your body responds to more strenuous forms of activity and a higher volume of exercise. Unfortunately, some women will skip Phase 2 altogether (or only spend a brief amount of time here) and proceed directly to Phase 3, as they are driven by their desire or perhaps an external pressure (e.g. sponsorship) to resume training as soon as possible. This is where the "mental battle" comes into play, especially since it is not uncommon for your brain to be ready before your body. Competitive triathlete, coach and mother of 2, Jessica Adam can relate to this. Despite her motivation and desire to start a more structured and intense training program, she was surprised how much physical recovery she needed after the birth of her first child. "Although I was looking forward to settling back into my training routine, I was shocked to find that I was completely winded after walking 1 kilometre," says Adam. "Your mind goes to a whole different place than

> **We Are Not Supermoms**
>
> "I think that there is a tendency for active women, including myself, to have higher expectations of ourselves and to assume that we can bounce back sooner," explains Deborah Moore, who has coached athletes in their postpartum period. "Given that we might have some advantages over the non-athletic person, we perhaps overestimate our body's superpowers and underestimate the lingering effects of pregnancy and childbirth. As a result, we may end up thinking that we are ready to exercise sooner than we are actually ready to. By letting our minds do the talking, we end up putting our bodies at risk."
> *Deborah Moore, coach, Ironman triathlete and mother of 3*

your body after pregnancy; learning to get your mind and body on the same page is key."

Looking at Your Readiness

Not sure if you are ready to take it up a notch? Although you cannot rely purely on time (e.g. I will start exercising in 2 weeks), there are several considerations that can help make this decision:

- Do you have any medical and physical restrictions to exercising right now?
- Have you been seen by your doctor or midwife postpartum?
- Will you listen to how your body responds to exercise?
- Are you exercising for the right reasons?

Consideration #1: Medical and Physical Restrictions
Although different sources may vary with their description, the following medical and physical considerations are commonly referred to when evaluating one's readiness to exercise:

- Wait until all soreness in the perineum region is gone, especially if you had an episiotomy.
- Wait until any heavy and bright red bleeding stops.
- Wait until you no longer experience heavy pelvic pressure.

Put more simply, Dr. James Clapp summarizes these restrictions in the following manner in his book *Exercising Through Your Pregnancy*: "...if it does not hurt or cause you to bleed, then it is ok." If you experience any of the above signs or symptoms after exercising, you may want to consider waiting a few days before trying the activity again.

Consideration #2: Postpartum Check Up
It is commonly suggested that you hold off exercising until you have seen your doctor or midwife, usually around 6 weeks postpartum. Up until then your body is at its greatest risk for complications, such as anemia, blood clots and wound infections (if you had a caesarean). During this routine check-up, your doctor or midwife examines the extent of your healing and determines:

- Has your uterus returned to its normal size?
- Have your cuts and tears healed properly?
- Are your pelvic floor muscles weak?

Your doctor might also order blood work to monitor your hormone levels, hemoglobin and iron stores. Another reason for the recommended 6-week waiting period is that your overall level of comfort will likely be much greater at this point. Some women have explained that "things suddenly felt different" around this time. Tania Jones, one of Canada's top marathoners and mother of 2, sensed that at about 4 weeks postpartum, her pelvis "shifted back to a pre-pregnancy position", which seemed to alleviate her back pain.

This is not to say that you must wait until you have seen your doctor for your postpartum check-up before initiating an exercise routine. In fact, many women started to exercise before seeing their doctor. The point that we want to emphasize is that it takes time for your body to heal and that the chance of complications is greatest during the first 6-week period. Erring on the side of caution and holding off on exercising may be a wise choice if you suspect that your body is not quite ready yet.

Consideration #3: Re-Connecting with Your Body
It now becomes increasingly important to be in tune with your body and to see how it handles your workouts on a regular basis. However, paying attention to how your body responds may be harder than you think, at least initially. Let's face it - your body has been through a lot and has changed in many ways. It is not surprising that your body might feel a bit foreign to you. In addition, you likely have not done a more strenuous workout in quite some time and therefore, the activity in itself may feel a bit awkward at first.

So, how do you distinguish between the typical soreness that you may experience following a new type of activity versus a "not quite right" response? Although it varies from woman to woman, you can use your past experience as an athlete and let your intuition tell you when the symptoms are atypical. Listen to your inner voice and, when in doubt, be cautious and scale back on your workout. "Simply getting the go-ahead from your doctor to exercise is not enough; if the exercise does not feel right, avoid doing it," suggests Trish Del Sorbo, former owner and director of Baby and Me Fitness.

The following describes some of the ways women realized they had taken on more than their bodies could handle at the time:

- *I felt like my insides were going to fall out.*
- *My pelvis area felt sore and bruised after the workout.*
- *Every time I tried to pick up the pace a little bit, it felt like my pelvis would break.*
- *Everything felt like it was sinking in my body.*
- *I just had too many aches and pains following my workouts.*

Paying attention to your body also means giving yourself permission NOT to exercise through pain during a workout. Although you might have been accustomed to doing so in your pre-pregnancy training days, your body may simply not be ready for this yet. You might also find it helpful to exercise on your own, rather than with a group or a training partner. Doing so allows you to devote your attention to how you are feeling, rather than getting caught up in a conversation with your training partner and exercising longer than anticipated, or letting your competitive nature take over and going harder than intended.

Consideration #4: Your Motivation

Understanding your reasons to start exercising again can help ensure that your motivation is stemming from a feeling of "want" rather than a feeling of "should". For instance:

- Are you rushing to start exercising because you are dissatisfied with your body and want to lose the weight as soon as possible?
- Do you feel pressured by yourself or others, such as your partner, coach or sponsor to start training as soon as possible?
- Do you enjoy exercising and look forward to settling back into a routine?

> **Running for the Right Reason**
>
> Stephanie Summers ran a 10K race 6 weeks after her baby was born. Although she did not realize it at the time, a key factor in her decision to run the race was the pressure she placed on herself to resume competing. "Because my sponsors were hosting the race, I felt like I owed it to the company to run the race," says Summers. "Looking back, I realize that it was too soon and that my body simply was not ready for this intensity."
> *Stephanie Summers, competitive runner, triathlete and mother of 2*

154

Exercising due to a sense of obligation will likely leave you feeling disappointed, frustrated and may even lead to negative feelings toward a sport that you once had a passion for. Perhaps more importantly, it may also lead to injuries and further setbacks. Upon reflection, you may decide that you are not quite ready for Phase 2. If so, that is fine. What is most important is being honest with yourself. Have faith that when the timing is right for you, you will be raring to go!

Getting Started

Assuming that you are now ready to start exercising in a consistent manner and engage in more strenuous types of exercise, the question then becomes, "how much is too much"? Unfortunately, there is no simple answer - it differs from woman to woman, and is based on your previous level of fitness, your overall pregnancy experience, your emotional wellness and your body's current state of readiness. Furthermore, it is not necessarily a matter of repeating the routine you did during pregnancy. For instance, if you were swimming 4 days a week for 30 minutes prior to giving birth, you may now find that this is too exhausting, especially if your sleep is often interrupted. A more appropriate exercise routine might be to start with 2-3 days per week for 15 minutes at a time. Although we have cautioned doing too much, too soon, it is worthwhile to mention that doing too little is also not advisable. Doing too little may leave you feeling dissatisfied and can deprive you of the many benefits of exercising. It all comes down to finding the right balance for you. Sometimes this takes some trial and error. The following points provide further guidance when trying to determine "how much is too much":

- Exercising right now should be about personal time, enjoyment and relaxation, not regaining your previous fitness level as soon as possible.
- Exercise should make you sweat a little, while at the same time, make you feel good.
- Be consistent in your aim to exercise several times a week but don't get too caught up with having a firm schedule (e.g. I must exercise on Monday, Wednesday and Friday). Rather, do something active when it is convenient for you and when the opportunity presents itself.
- Be flexible. Your family is still settling into a routine, thereby making your schedule unpredictable. Being consistent is as easy

as getting out the door for 15 minutes of exercise, rather than not getting out at all! The point is to do something active and let your body become familiar with this new routine.

- If exercise leaves you very stiff, sore and fatigued (for greater than 48 hours) or if it is not enjoyable, it may be a sign that you are doing too much. Ease up on your workout or try a different type of exercise.
- Avoid the temptation to analyze your performance level. Instead, enjoy the moment and celebrate knowing that you have succeeded in making exercise a priority and you are on the road to consistency.
- Modify your exercise if you experience any of the signs of overexertion listed in Table 15.0.

Spending enough time in this phase, as opposed to rushing into a more structured, intense, goal-orientated training plan (Phase 3) will help to ensure that as your body adjusts to its "new normal", you will start to increase your training and overall fitness foundation. By "testing out the waters" with some consistent training and more strenuous workouts, you will likely suffer less injuries in the long term. Consider for a moment the new mom who wants to start running again. Despite feeling ready, she may be unaware of some of the more subtle changes to her body. Her running gait may have altered slightly during her pregnancy due to her added weight, the flattening of her feet and the widening of her hips. Her core may not be as strong as it was before pregnancy and her upper back may be sore from always holding her baby. Such changes may result in less than optimal running mechanics, which over time, can lead to injuries – especially if she increases her running mileage too quickly and introduces speed workouts before her body is ready. Getting injured

Everything Was Fine...at First

I began running when my son was about 2 months old. I started off slowly and gradually built up my tolerance to 40 minutes, 3 times a week. But every time I tried running beyond this, I would experience deep soreness in my left hip. It was very frustrating and forced me to cut back a lot on my running and spend more time cycling and swimming. Perhaps if I would have sought treatment and focused on strength work early on, much of this could have been avoided.

Zoe Webster, mountain biker, runner and mother of 2

and having to take more time off is probably the last thing she will want after curbing her activity level for the last 9 months.

To further illustrate our point, consider the following biking analogy: After having the misfortune of crashing on your bike, you probably would not think twice about having your bike checked out by a bike mechanic. Otherwise, you know that you risk the chance of it not working properly, especially as you begin to log more miles on your bike. Why not take the same proactive measures with your own body, given what it has been through? You cannot always assume that your body will heal on its own and return to its exact pre-pregnancy state.

If you are serious about getting back into your sport or if you want to train harder, consider seeing a qualified health or sports professional, such as a physiotherapist or a kinesiologist for a thorough head-to-toe assessment. They can help determine your body's functional readiness to handle the specific movements and characteristics of your sport. Do you have any muscle weaknesses or imbalances? Do you have adequate core strength and balance? Investing the time upfront (before progressing to Phase 3) to identify potential problems can save you from experiencing any injuries or setbacks later on.

Strengthen That Body
Finally, this brings us to the last important consideration for Phase 2, which is the incorporation of strength work into your training routine. This recommendation applies to all new moms, regardless of whether or not you have gotten a thorough head-to-toe assessment that may identify any muscle imbalances or weaknesses. As your body starts to adjust to its "new normal", more physical changes are going to occur. Introducing strength training at this point in time may help to lessen the pregnancy effects on your body as it adjusts to such changes, while potentially minimizing the risk of injuries as you return to your sport. Fortunately, this does not mean that you need to join a gym and spend hours in the weight room in order to become strong. In fact, a little can go a long way! To start, try a few body-weighted exercises every 2-3 days; they can be done in the convenience of your home, while your little one is napping. For example: try doing push-ups, triceps dips, squats and lunges. You can start with 1 set of 10-15 repetitions for the first few weeks and then add another set as tolerated. Refer to Appendix 4 "Strengthening Exercises for the Pregnant Athlete" for detailed explanations regarding form and technique.

Jennifer Faraone & Dr. Carol Ann Weis

Summary

After being patient and letting your body heal, you will find that, over time, you will become stronger and want to engage in some type of moderate exercise – including more strenuous forms of weight bearing activities, several times a week. It is not about striving for peak fitness or losing your baby weight as soon as possible. Rather, the goals are to promote fitness, offer enjoyment and provide you with a sense of control again. There are several considerations that can help assess your readiness for Phase 2. These include the extent to which your body has healed, the results of your postpartum check-up with your doctor or midwife, your ability to re-connect and listen to your body's response to exercise and your reasons and/or motivation for wanting to exercise again.

Chapter 17

PHASE 3: YOUR STRUCTURED TRAINING PROGRAM

How do I plan a weekly training schedule when everyday is so unpredictable?
What should my plan include?
How do I juggle motherhood and training?

One, Two, THREE...GO!
Were you successful with exercising consistently several times a week? Are you feeling strong and healthy? Are you motivated to train for a specific goal or event? If you have answered yes to these questions – congratulations, you are now ready for Phase 3 and to initiate a more structured, intense and goal-oriented training plan (Figure 17.0). Although establishing a solid training program can be a bit more challenging for you as a new mom, rest assured that with some simple planning and perseverance it will all come together.

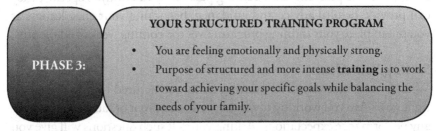

PHASE 3:

YOUR STRUCTURED TRAINING PROGRAM
- You are feeling emotionally and physically strong.
- Purpose of structured and more intense **training** is to work toward achieving your specific goals while balancing the needs of your family.

Figure 17.0: Phase 3: Your Structured Training Program

Once again, you will notice that we have not made specific reference to timing (e.g. I will start to train at 3 months postpartum). There are other variables that should be considered, including your body's readiness, your level of motivation and your personal circumstances (e.g. the availability of childcare or inadequate sleep) that will either facilitate or hinder your training. Rather, we recommend developing your training program based on the following components:

- Realistic, achievable and meaningful goals
- A blend of desired activities including sport-specific workouts, strength training, cross-training and rest activities
- Creative strategies that work for you and your family, so that you can be a mom who finds the time to train
- Periodic "check-ins" to assess how things are going

Creating Positive Expectations

Jessica Adam, a competitive athlete, mother and coach with Lifesport, explains that a large part of what she does while coaching (especially to new moms) is providing support and helping manage expectations in a positive manner. "For many athletic moms, it comes as a surprise that being a mom is really 24/7 and that it can be hard to switch off the parenting hat when it comes time to train. I let them know that it is okay to miss workouts due to parenting requirements," explains Adam. "As needed, we work together to revisit their goals and training. Providing this support and letting them know that I can relate to what they are going through, is just as important as giving them a detailed training plan."

Jessica Adam, triathlete, coach and mother of 2

Ideally, your training program is developed with input from your coach, exercise professionals, training partners and family. Together, they can provide helpful advice and guidance, becoming your cheerleaders as you put in place your training program over the coming weeks and months.

Setting Your Goals

What is your motivation for starting a more structured training program right now? Are you working toward a particular event or race? Do you have any performance expectations? Asking yourself such questions will give you a chance to reflect on your own level of motivation and specific interests, which in turn will help shape your plan. You may come to realize that your interests have changed from your pre-pregnancy training days. For instance, prior to pregnancy, you may have competed in Olympic distance triathlons (1.5K swim - 40K bike - 10K run), whereas now, you may be interested in sprint distance duathlons (2K run - 20K bike - 5K run), as it is more achievable to train fewer hours and to focus on 2 sports instead of 3.

If your heart is set on a particular performance goal (e.g. running a 10K race under 40 minutes), you may want to be cautious with attaching a specific timeframe for reaching this particular goal (e.g. in 6 months). There are many variables that can influence how soon you regain your fitness, so you may only be setting yourself up for frustration and disappointment. Focusing instead on progressive and achievable goals may be more appropriate. For instance, a more suitable goal might be to compete in 3 consecutive 10K races, while aiming to run each one faster. Alternatively, you may decide to focus initially on a particular aspect of your sport, such as perfecting your swim stroke, knowing that you can always work on your speed later on.

Finally, your goals should take into account both your short and your long-term objectives. Dr. Julia Alleyne, a sport and exercise physician, asks her athletes to consider training in terms of priorities. Rather than focusing on the next event, she encourages the athlete to think about what is the most important event, as this can help set more realistic expectations with your training. Is your goal to qualify for the Boston Marathon next year? If so, then training for the 10K event that is a month away may not be ideal, given that your goal is a

---

My Story: Taking It One Race at a Time!

I found it hard to gauge my fitness after the birth of my son Dominic. I therefore found it more helpful and motivating to run several 5K races in a row, with a goal of running each one faster, as opposed to aiming for a particular time (e.g. under 21 minutes).

My first race was a local community run, about 2 months postpartum. This race gave me a sense of my current fitness level. I ran a second race about a month later and was able to run a minute faster. I ran my third race a few months later and shaved another 90 seconds off my time. And finally, at 10 months postpartum, I had reached a new personal best.

Jennifer Faraone, co-author, competitive duathlete and runner, mother of 2

Hard Work Pays Off

Prior to getting pregnant, I had been trying to get hired by the Fire Department – which involved passing the same vigorous physical test as my male counterparts. Now that my baby was born, I was eager to apply again. But I knew that the physical test would be no easy feat - the first time I hit the gym I could only do 1 sit up! But I persevered, hired 2 personal trainers and 6 months later, I passed the test!

Allison Chisholm, triathlete and mother of 2

161

year away. Is it worth the risk of training too aggressively, too soon and becoming injured?

Will there be times when you are discouraged with your training and feel that your goals are out of reach? Probably and that is normal! Although it can be difficult to predict exactly when it will happen, trust that with enough patience, effort and commitment – your goals will be reached.

Designing Your Training Plan

After choosing your goals and expectations, the next step is to develop some form of schedule or plan that works toward achieving them. It is preferable to develop a customized plan, as opposed to simply using your pre-pregnancy one or replicating someone else's plan, as it will take into consideration your current lifestyle, training history, activity levels during your pregnancy, postpartum recovery, motivations and training goals. More specifically, a customized training plan will benefit you by:

- Providing a clear sense of purpose and direction.
- Promoting a blend of activities that complement each other and work toward a common goal.
- Facilitating gradual progressions of volume and intensity in a safe manner.
- Reducing the risk of injury and overtraining.
- Providing motivation.

> **Coach's Corner**
> When one of my athletes feels ready to resume her training postpartum, I typically will have her start running with low mileage at an easy pace. The approach is similar to that of an athlete who is just coming back following an injury - mileage build-up needs to be gradual. I prefer waiting several months before adding intensity, as she is most likely training through a fair amount of fatigue from erratic sleep. It is best to build an aerobic base without taxing the system with intense workouts. After 3 months, I may add 1 interval session per week, followed by a second one several months later.
> *Nicole Stevenson, former professional runner and coach*

Your training plan can be as detailed as you like. It may be written on a piece of paper and intended for your eyes only, or it may be something more formal that was developed with your coach and reviewed on a weekly basis. The key is that your plan has been well thought out and tailored to your specific needs. In turn, it will maximize your enjoyment, optimize your performance and minimize any setbacks.

The following steps can assist with designing your plan:

1. Identify the types of workouts that you would like to accomplish in a given week. Ideally, this would include your sport-specific activities, some form of cross training, full-body and core strengthening activities and rest. Engaging in a variety of workouts will help keep the plan interesting while minimizing the risk of injury.

2. Schedule the workouts in a practical manner. This might include the more traditional method of scheduling them according to the days of the week or on a rotating 7-10 day schedule. Alternatively, you may find the "checklist approach" (discussed next) to be particularly helpful at first. Regardless of the method, avoid scheduling hard workouts back-to-back.

3. Incorporate a "build" approach that allows for a gradual progression of volume and/or intensity. For instance, your weekly volume of mileage is increased by 5-10% for 2-3 consecutive weeks followed by a reduction in the following week. Such an approach minimizes the risk of doing too much, too soon and will give your body more time to adapt to the increasing demands of your workouts. If this is too aggressive, simply keep your mileage the same until you feel ready to progress.

> **The Joy of Napping**
>
> One of the best tips I received to balance training and motherhood was napping. Napping gave me the energy to care for my children, to train and to keep the house in order. To this day, 1:00 pm remains my quiet time, which I strongly value. If I am sleeping and recovering properly from training, I may only need 20 minutes. However, other days it may be longer. On those particular days, dinner may be thrown together a little quicker than normal!
>
> *Krista DuChene, professional runner and mother of 3*

4. Schedule a day (or more) of rest and actually use it. Although you may have been used to training every day prior to pregnancy, your body may appreciate the additional down time as you balance your current lifestyle.

5. As necessary, seek assistance from a coach that has experience working with athletic moms. Not only can they help with the logistics of your plan, they may also be more understanding of your new lifestyle.

The Checklist Approach

As a new mom, you might appreciate a training plan that offers the most flexibility with scheduling your workouts, especially when every day is different and it can be difficult to adhere to a schedule. The checklist approach can be helpful in such circumstances, as it removes the need to plan too far in advance and takes into account what is happening on any given day. Developing your checklist is easy and can be done by yourself or with a coach, using the following steps:

1. Identify the minimum number and types of workouts that you want to accomplish during a particular week. For instance: 3 runs, a bike, a yoga and a strength session. Be as descriptive as you can. For instance: 1 moderate pace run for 45 minutes, 1 relaxed run for 70 minutes and 1 speed session for 60 minutes.
2. Decide whether you want to use a ranking system to help prioritize the workouts. "A" workouts are your "must do" activities and "B" activities are "nice to do" ones.
3. Place the activities in a simple table format, as illustrated in the following table (Table 17.0).
4. Every morning (or the night before), decide which activity, if any, you want to perform on that particular day. Your decision is based on several factors, such as how much time you have, childcare availability, your energy levels and how your baby is feeling. Avoid doing 2 strenuous workouts in a row.
5. Keep track of the completed workouts by writing down helpful information, such as how you felt during the workout and whether the workout went as expected.

Table 17.0: Checklist Approach

Week:			
Planned Activities	Rank	Done	Comments
Speed run: 3x1K repeats plus warm up and cool down 60 minutes	A		
Easy pace run 70 minutes	B		
Moderate pace run 45 minutes	A		
Yoga DVD 45 minutes	B		
Upper and lower body and core strength work 1 hour	A		
Indoor cycling 30 minutes	B		

As the days (and your child) become more predictable, switching to a calendar format training plan may be more feasible.

Balancing It All

You identified your goals and developed your training plan. So, now you are all set to go, right? Not necessarily! As you have probably come to realize, being a mom is anything but simple, straightforward and predictable. There are numerous factors that can limit your ability to follow through with your intended training plan. The success of your training is based on how

> **Where My Training Takes Place**
> My training is quite different now that I have 2 children. Each day is full of so many unpredictable variables (e.g. kids waking up early, disrupted naps and crankiness), that I no longer work with a coach or follow a structured training plan. In fact, 90% of my training now happens on a spin bike in our living room during nap time or while pushing the running stroller on paved paths and country roads.
> *Kelley Cullen, XTERRA triathlete and mother of 2*

you handle competing priorities and "less-than-ideal" circumstances, while minimizing the disruption that training has on your family. In other words, it is about finding the best way to balance your training and motherhood. Sometimes figuring out this balance takes a bit of time and creativity. Jessica Zelinka, a Canadian Olympic heptathlete, 100m hurdler and mother of 1, recalls the struggle she faced at first. "The biggest stressor for me postpartum was finding how to strike a balance between training and being a mom. Training was the easy part, as it was more predictable than my daughter."

These competing priorities and less-than-ideal circumstances come in a variety of forms and may include:

- Your child not sleeping throughout the night.
- Your child not napping consistently during the day.
- Your child experiencing separation anxiety and crying a lot when you leave the room.
- Your child feeding on demand.
- Your child refusing a bottle.
- Your child frequently getting sick.
- Your other children craving your attention.
- Not having family close by that can help with childcare.
- Your spouse travelling a lot for work.
- Your training group meeting at inconvenient times.

Making It Work for You and Your Family

Many of the athletic moms who have remained committed to their training have something in common: a knack for figuring out how to make it work for themselves and for their family. After all, if your plan does not work for the entire family, your training is likely not going to go as expected, nor will it provide you with the satisfaction you anticipated.

For professional triathlete Tara Norton, "making it work" means sitting down with her husband every week and scheduling her workouts around her child's activities and her husband's work commitments. For Belinda Bain, who manages to train at least 10 hours a week, on top of working full-time as a lawyer and raising her children, it means focusing on the things that matter most, like spending time together as a family after her morning workouts and letting go of some of the more mundane activities. For Allison Chisholm, who needs to be creative when trying to log a high volume of training (both she and her husband are firefighters and work shiftwork), she finds ways to involve her family in her workouts so that her training becomes a family affair.

The point is that there will always be something that gets in the way of completing a workout and sticking to a plan. That is the reality that all athletic moms face at some point or another. What sets apart the mom who is able to stick to her plan (versus the one that does not) may simply be credited to the way in which she is able to identify and address these challenges. For instance, you may decide to hold off training for a few weeks until your baby learns to drink from a bottle and is not as dependent on you for feeding. You may decide that training with your previous group is no longer convenient and will look for a new group that meets during the day, closer to your home. Finding an alternate solution to training is better than doing nothing at all!

Getting your groove back may also require a slight shift in the way you approach your training and how you perceive yourself as an athlete. It is not the number of hours that you spend exercising, the intensity of your workout or whom you train with that defines you as an athlete. You are still an athlete, but how you go about your training may change now that you are also a mother. Such was the case for Danelle Kabush, professional XTERRA triathlete and mother of 2. "I now focus more on the quality than the quantity of training, as I do not want to be gone from my kids for hours every day," explains Kabush. "My racing expectations have not changed in that I do not expect any less of myself. I still work just as hard as ever, maybe just a few less junk hours."

Furthermore, your level of confidence can also have an impact on how you approach your training. According to Alleyne, that may be easier for the professional athlete who has more experience with respect to coming back strong following a period of recovery. Such athletes have a small advantage in that they worked with sports psychologists on how to instil confidence in their body during performance and recovery periods. This level of confidence can help them to focus on the appropriate amount of training at any given time; they know that the foundation is there and are not afraid of losing their fitness. Not having such confidence can either put you at risk of doing too much exercise too soon, out of fear of losing your fitness or not doing enough, out of fear of the unknown.

So keep in mind that with a little creativity, patience and confidence, you *will* be able to balance motherhood and training. Getting your groove back *will* happen.

Periodic Check-Ins

Once your plan is well underway, it is a good idea to periodically "check-in" with yourself and reflect on your training. For instance:

- Is the plan working out as intended for you and your family?
- Are you getting the enjoyment and satisfaction you anticipated?
- Are you able to follow the plan most of the time?
- Are you healthy and injury free?

If you answer "no" to any of these questions, it can be a sign that your training plan requires modification. You may need to revisit your goals and modify them slightly or incorporate shorter but more efficient workouts. Nicole Stevenson, the coach referred to in the sidebar "Coaches Corner", stresses the need for honesty and awareness when assessing how the athletes are doing. "Now is not the time to suck it up and push through niggles or pains, as her body and lifestyle are adjusting to so many things," explains Stevenson. "After starting their training plans, many new moms find that they have less time and energy than anticipated; it is important to frequently revisit and tweak the expectations and the plan." Refer to the Table 17.1 for signs of overtraining and how to manage.

Table 17.1: Signs of Overtraining

Overtraining is a risk that all athletes face, especially when trying to find the right level of training. Although it can appear differently from one person to another, the following are some of the more common signs and symptoms:

- Decreased physical performance
- Increased aches and pains
- Greater number of injuries
- Increased resting heart rate
- Greater bouts of sickness
- Slower recovery between workouts
- Increased perceived exertion
- Loss of enthusiasm or motivation to exercise
- Changes in sleep patterns
- Loss of appetite

If you suspect that you are overtraining, it is important to back off and allow for a few days of rest. As you feel better, take the time to re-evaluate your training plan and decide what needs adjusting. You may need to experiment a bit before finding the right balance between rest and activity.

Upon reflection, you may come to the realization that a structured training plan may not be suitable for you right now. Balancing motherhood and training is challenging and you are no less of an athlete should you choose to postpone your training. Be proud of yourself for making such a difficult decision and trust that your time to shine as an athlete will come.

Can Pregnancy Make You a Better Athlete?

Is there any truth to the notion that female athletes achieve higher performance levels after having children? The idea first came from reported stories about European athletes in the early 20th century who would intentionally get pregnant in order to boost their performance. Despite limited studies, there are many anecdotal stories from athletes themselves supporting this idea.

From a physiological standpoint, there is some truth to this idea, as many of the changes that occur to a woman's body during pregnancy, including an elevated heart rate and increased blood volume, mimics what normally happens when a non-pregnant person trains consistently over a period of time. However, it remains to be seen whether some of the reported improvements (observed most often with elite athletes) are more directly linked to how soon a woman returns to training postpartum and her accessibility to certain resources, such as a coach, personal trainer or physiotherapist. Many women do report feeling mentally stronger after giving birth, which ultimately can also lead to better performances. So, while achieving personal bests after giving birth is a possibility, it is not a guarantee.

Summary
Starting a training program can be hard for anyone, let alone a new mom who is juggling competing priorities and settling into a new routine. Identifying realistic goals, designing a customized training program that accommodates your personal circumstances and periodically checking in with your body's response, will, nonetheless, make your postpartum comeback that much easier and enjoyable for you and your family.

Chapter 18

THE BREASTFEEDING ATHLETE

Does training have an effect on my breast milk?
Will breastfeeding limit my ability to train optimally?
What can I do to make breastfeeding easier?

Making the "Breast" Decision for You and Your Baby

Breastfeeding is a wonderful way to bond with your child, while providing an abundance of benefits to you both. It is for these reasons that many leading sources, including the Canadian Pediatric Society, Dietitians of Canada, Health Canada, the Academy of Breastfeeding Medicine and the World Health Organization, recommend exclusive breastfeeding for the first 6 months of life and continued breastfeeding with complementary foods for up to 2 years and beyond.

The decision to breastfeed is yours. There is no right or wrong answer as it is based on your own personal circumstances. Although it is

> ### Sprouting Your Child's Inner Athlete
> You may already know that breastfeeding provides your baby with numerous health benefits, such as protection from infections and diseases, less chance of developing eczema and less likelihood of obesity. You may even know that breastfeeding provides you with health benefits as well, such as lowering your risk of breast and ovarian cancer. But did you know that breastfeeding may also influence your child's athletic abilities? A recent study found that adolescents who were breastfed as a child had stronger leg muscles and were better able to perform jumping exercises, in comparison to those who were not breastfed. Published in the Journal of Nutrition, the authors Artero et al. (2010) also found that the longer the children were breastfed, the stronger their leg muscles were. Although there is not enough information to say whether these kids went on to become better athletes, it is, nevertheless, an interesting finding regarding the benefits of breastfeeding.

often referred to as "the natural thing to do", do not be surprised if you encounter challenges along the way. What you may not realize is that breastfeeding is actually a learned skill; for many new moms, their first real experience with breastfeeding is when their baby arrives. Dallas Parsons, International Board Certified Lactation Consultant, dietitian and founder of Best Start Breastfeeding & Nutrition, explains that there are a variety of factors that can make breastfeeding somewhat easier – or harder! Such factors may include the positioning of your child when breastfeeding, your anxiety or calorie and fluid intake, to name a few. If you have difficulties, Parsons reassures that most breastfeeding challenges can be overcome with proper guidance and support. "Each breastfeeding mother and baby has their own rhythm and when this is recognized and respected, things often go well."

Many times, the influence of such factors on breastfeeding is what leads new athletic moms to ask additional questions, especially with regard to exercising. *Does training interfere with breastfeeding? Are more calories required to maintain an adequate milk supply? What can be done to make exercising more comfortable, given the larger (and sometimes sore) breasts?* Fortunately, the take-away message is positive: you CAN train while breastfeeding. Furthermore, it is often not the exercise, per say, that may cause challenges with breastfeeding; rather, it could be certain outcomes from your training, such as dehydration, rapid and excessive weight loss and exhaustion that could negatively influence the ease with which you breastfeed. In other words, any difficulty you encounter is not necessarily attributed to your training. Therefore, it is important to step back and consider the other factors that may be interfering with breastfeeding.

> **A Declining Rate**
>
> A recent study of breastfeeding for first-time mothers by Toronto Public Health showed that only 17.6 % of the mothers who initiated breastfeeding at the time of birth continued to breastfeed exclusively at 6 months postpartum. A variety of reasons were suggested for this declining rate, including the need for more information on the benefits and the management of breastfeeding.

It should be noted that some of these factors, such as the proper positioning of your baby or the various health-related conditions that could have an effect on breastfeeding, are beyond the scope of this book and will not be discussed here. Rather, the focus of this chapter is to discuss breastfeeding in the context of exercise and share with you the information and strategies that research and clinical experts and athletic moms have shared to enhance the breastfeeding experience for you and your baby.

What the Studies Show

There are several studies that have looked at exercise and breastfeeding, and their results are encouraging. For instance:

- Exercise, by itself, does not negatively affect the volume and quality of your breast milk.
- Your baby's weight is not directly affected by your training. Rather, the weight becomes more of an issue if your calorie intake is too low and affects your milk supply.
- There may be a brief and temporary increase of lactic acid in your breast milk when you exercise at maximal intensity for longer durations (as opposed to exercising at a lower intensity). However, this increase does not impact the nutritional value of the milk and usually disappears within the first hour following exercise. There are differing views about whether a higher level of lactic acid slightly affects the taste of the milk.
- You lose approximately 200mg of calcium per day when breastfeeding, which translates to 3-9% of bone mineral density loss during the course of 6 months. Your bone mass usually returns to normal levels once you stop breastfeeding. New research shows that resistance and aerobic exercise while breastfeeding can help reduce this amount of bone density loss.

These finding should provide reassurance that you can breastfeed while training; however, research is only part of the answer. What do other subject matter experts – including athletics moms – have to say? Once again, the findings are positive.

What the Athletic Moms Say

Many of the moms we interviewed did not experience any difficulties with breastfeeding while ramping up their training. However, a few struggled to maintain an adequate milk supply. Similarly, some moms found that their babies would happily nurse following an intense workout, whereas a small number of moms found their babies to be fussy during these feedings. Why such differences?

Once again, these differences speak to the fact that individual experiences with all aspects of motherhood vary and breastfeeding is no exception. That being said, it is encouraging to note that most of the women interviewed were successful in following through with their intentions to breastfeed. Although it may not have been easy at first and sometimes required assistance from others, the take away message is that they *were able* to breastfeed:

> **The Breastfeeding Marathon**
>
> If there was an ultramarathon for breastfeeding, I am the champion. I breastfed for 7 years, 8 months and 5 days. That's 2807 consecutive days of breastfeeding for just 2 children. I loved breastfeeding for its convenience and how wonderful and connected it made me and the kids feel. I didn't need to pack formula and milk was always available. My children didn't mind if I had just finished running - a sweaty breast still gives good milk. If we were having a stressful day, those good hormones from nursing relaxed both of us.
> *Jennifer Young, triathlete and mother of 2*

- The first few weeks of breastfeeding were difficult for both of us. But with a little perseverance and help from a lactation consultant, I managed to gain more confidence and it became an enjoyable and relaxing part of my day. My second and third children were much easier to breastfeed, as I had mastered the technique. *Karen Soos, marathon runner, mother of 3*

- I learned how important it was to ensure the baby latched on properly from the beginning and I was able to breastfeed each of my boys for 6-8 months. Nothing can replace the bonding and serenity that comes with breastfeeding. *Lucia Mahoney, runner, mother of 3*

- Although it took a few days to get the hang of it, I had no problems

> **Tough but Doable**
>
> Breastfeeding is tough. Trying to breastfeed and exercise is tougher and requires patience, timing and determination. But it can be done. The first few weeks were quite uncomfortable and I had to purchase larger exercising bras and pump prior to working out to relieve some of the pressure. Trying to arrange a run with friends at first was difficult, as my son was not on a schedule. The length of my runs was therefore based on how long I felt my child could go in between feeds. But by 3 months the engorgement subsided, my son's feeding became more predictable and breastfeeding became relatively easy.
> *Sharlene Cobain, runner and mother of 2*

breastfeeding with all of my 3 children. *Fulvia Manarin, runner, mother of 3*

- I was initially anxious about breastfeeding, but with some practice and guidance from the lactation consultants, breastfeeding turned out to be a wonderful experience. I nursed each of my 3 girls until they were 14 months old. *Alisa Bridgman, runner and triathlete, mother of 3*

- I really loved nursing. It was hard, but it was a priority for me because I believed in its importance. *Christiane Tremblay, triathlete, mother of 4*

Boosting Breastfeeding Through Better Nutrition

It can be common for new moms, especially athletic ones, to consume an insufficient amount of calories when breastfeeding. There are multiple reasons for this, such as restricting calorie intake in an effort to lose the extra weight, a lack of awareness of the required calorie intake, a preoccupation with attending to your newborn and simply forgetting to eat. "Finding the time to eat properly can be tricky, especially since it is easy to get caught up in the breastfeeding/diaper changing /caring for baby routine and neglecting myself," explains Sharlene Cobain, an elite runner and mother of 2. However, not consuming enough calories on a regular basis can be problematic if you are nursing, as this can reduce your milk supply. Dr. Julia Alleyne, a sport and exercise physician, explains that there needs to be a balance between the amount of calories consumed versus the amount of calories spent. This is why it is extremely important that you adjust your nutritional intake appropriately when you start to ramp up your training.

According to Taya Griffin, a breastfeeding consultant, new mothers typically need an additional 500 calories a day in the first couple of months of breastfeeding. However, this amount may change as your baby starts to eat solid food and/or is fed formula. It is important to note that this additional amount does not take into account the calories burned while exercising. Therefore, if you are exercising and breastfeeding, you will need to add even more calories to your daily intake. Griffin suggests assessing your level of exercise and increasing your calorie intake based on how vigorous your training is. You can also monitor your calorie intake by ensuring that the following conditions are met:

- Your baby appears happy and is gaining an appropriate amount of weight.
- You are not losing more than 1 lb. per week.
- You are not constantly feeling hungry or dehydrated.

As a nursing mom that exercises, you also need to pay attention to your fluid intake, as you may become dehydrated more easily. Dehydration can reduce your milk flow (i.e. the speed in which the milk comes out of your breast), causing your baby to fuss while breastfeeding. Increasing your fluid intake during the day, and perhaps more so when working out, can easily prevent this issue. Some signs of dehydration include an increase in thirst and dark coloured urine.

> **Another Reason to Eat Well**
>
> As a new mother, you may not be aware that you are on "the losing end" of nutrients when you breastfeed. "Many of the essential nutrients, including calcium and omega 3s, are going directly to your baby through your breast milk. This can leave your body deficient in these nutrients unless you increase their intake either through food or multivitamins," explains Jennifer Sygo, dietitian at Cleveland Clinic Canada. "Omega 3s are an important nutrient to increase when breastfeeding, as studies are now finding that a deficiency in this nutrient can increase one's chance of postpartum depression." Even more reason why eating well is important!

Breastfeeding Made Easier

There are additional factors that can allow for a more comfortable breastfeeding experience. Parsons recommends the following tactics when starting to exercise or when taking your training up a notch:

- *Breastfeed before exercising.* Nursing prior to working out will make your breasts feel considerably less heavy and more comfortable while exercising.
- *Try pumping.* If you are concerned about missing a feeding while exercising for a long period of time, try expressing your milk with a pump or with your hand and storing it in the fridge before heading out the door.
- *Relax.* If your child seems to fuss while breastfeeding immediately after your workout, wait a few minutes then try again. This fussiness could be due to a number of factors, including your own anxiety. This anxiety can result if your

adrenaline (from exercise) is still high and you are finding it hard to relax, or if there is a sense of urgency to nurse your child as quickly as possible. Such anxiety can affect your letdown and the ease in which your milk flows. Try taking a few deep breaths or a warm shower to help calm you and to facilitate your letdown.

- ***Invest in a supportive sports bra.*** Wearing a well-fitted bra is key to being comfortable. You want to ensure that the bra is not too tight, especially as your breasts start to engorge, as this could lead to blocked ducts in your breast. Blocked ducts can lead to mastitis, an infection in your breast that will make them sore and tender.

> **Breastfeeding and Race Bibs**
>
> I participated in my first triathlon 10 weeks postpartum. I did not let the fact that I was breastfeeding stop me; rather, I simply incorporated it into my race routine. After registering for the race and picking up my race bib, I found a quiet place to breastfeed, and then joined the others on the starting line. Everyone was happy – my baby was content with a full stomach and I was out there having a great time participating in the race.
>
> *Belinda Bain, cyclist and mother of 2*

- ***Remove your wet, sweaty bra right away.*** Hanging out in your sweaty clothes (where bacteria likes to grow) after a workout can also increase your chance of developing mastitis. Mastitis can also develop when bacteria enters the body through an opening in cracked nipples. Removing your wet sports bra as soon as possible, quickly wiping your breasts with a washcloth or wearing a bra made out of material that wicks away moisture can help to minimize the risk of infection.

Parsons also encourages women to set their goals when it comes to breastfeeding, just as one would do in training and then communicate their goals to people within their support network. "Many women have been creative in finding ways to breastfeed and exercise and the support of spouses and coaches can make this transition even easier," explains Parsons. Danelle Kabush, professional Xterra athlete and mother of 2, found the following strategy useful: "What helped us the most was investing in an electric breast pump and introducing a bottle when the timing was right. It took more time and required more organization (especially prior to a race), but it worked for us." If you are still encountering some challenges with breastfeeding, rest assured that help is available. For more information and support, try contacting your local public health unit, La Leche League (www.lllc.ca), or the International Board Certified Lactation Consultants (www.ilca.org).

Summary
As a new mom who is motivated to resume training and breastfeed your child, you will be happy to know that you can do both. Applying certain tactics, such as ensuring proper hydration and calorie intake, as well as scheduling feedings around the timing of your workout, will further facilitate your ability to breastfeed. If you do encounter challenges, keep in mind that there are numerous factors that can interfere with breastfeeding and it may not necessarily be related to your training. Seek help from a trained lactation consultant or other qualified professionals as necessary.

GOING THE EXTRA MILE

Chapter 19

EXPANDING YOUR SUPPORT TEAM

Do I simply have to "grin and bear" the many discomforts of pregnancy?
Is there a role for chiropractors, physiotherapists etc. during my pregnancy?
What can I do to maximize my comfort level, given the changes that my
body is going through?

Times Are Changing

Not that long ago, most people would have given little thought to their "pregnancy team". In fact, most women would have interacted almost inclusively with their doctor or midwife. There is no doubt that this person will be the most engaged during your pregnancy; after all, they are probably spending the most amount of time with you and monitoring the health of you and your baby. But in today's day and age, things are changing and more people are becoming involved in a woman's pregnancy. Part of this change is due to the growing number of professionals that are more readily available, such as doulas, fertility specialists, lactation consultants and so on. But part of this change is also due to our attitudes and beliefs regarding injury prevention and optimal health - not just for pregnancy but also for a greater sense of wellness overall. In fact, athletes are great advocates for taking an active approach to seeking care and treatment when a sports-related injury arises or when they want to prevent one from happening in the first place.

Network of Practitioners

There is a good chance that if you ask an athlete to refer a good sports medicine physician, physiotherapist or chiropractor, you will likely be given a name and contact information right there on the spot! In fact, many athletes will use a combination of different health care providers and other forms of complementary and alternative medicine (CAM) to minimize their risk of injury, treat nagging injuries and promote a healthy training season.

Although you may already have some form of support team that keeps you healthy as an athlete, you may not realize the role that such practitioners can play during your pregnancy. In fact, utilizing the services of your support team, in addition to your relationship with your obstetrician/midwife, can be a great adjunct to your overall prenatal and postnatal care, *especially* if you continue to be active. Your body is going through such tremendous changes and enlisting the help from your support team can help with the way that your body responds to such changes and maximize your comfort level. For example, you may have worked with a practitioner, other than

> **Your Support Team**
>
> As an athlete, you may have had your share of appointments with a variety of different practitioners to better help you prevent or manage injuries and ensure that you can perform your best on race day. We refer such a group of health care providers and other types of complementary and alternative medicine (CAM) as your "support team" and may include, but are not limited to, any of the following:
>
> | | |
> |---|---|
> | Sports medicine physician | Registered massage therapist |
> | Chiropractor | Physiotherapist |
> | Osteopath | Dietitian |
> | Nutritionist | Naturopath |
> | Homeopath | Chiropodist |
>
> Complementary refers to treatment given alongside conventional medicine, like an herbal supplement, whereas alternative medicine refers to treatment that is not considered conventional, like seeing an osteopath or acupuncturist.

your doctor, to treat and manage certain health related issues such as a physiotherapist to strengthen your leg muscles after a surgery, or a dietitian to help manage your diabetes through adequate food intake. These same practitioners can help manage and prevent some of the discomforts and changes associated with pregnancy. In fact, utilizing the services of your support team can potentially make a significant difference in your overall pregnancy experience - and in some cases, could mean the difference between continuing to exercise or not! Remember - do not shy away from telling your primary health care provider when receiving care from any of these practitioners. Together, they can work toward ensuring that you have a healthy and active pregnancy.

Supporting You During Your Pregnancy
As discussed in the chapter "The Pregnant Athlete's Body", your body is undergoing some major changes during this time. Changes include the more obvious musculoskeletal ones (e.g. the protruding abdomen, increased breast size and rounded shoulders), as well as the not-so-obvious ones (e.g. hormonal fluctuations). Although many of the changes are inevitable with pregnancy, it does not mean that you should simply put on a brave face and tolerate the discomfort. You can have some control over how much they affect you. This is where your network of practitioners, or your "support team", can provide some relief. If they helped you in the past with your training, why not let them also support you now?

Although the specific types of services varies according to the type of practitioner and their individual scope of practice, your support team could potentially provide the following benefits during your pregnancy by:

- Lessening or preventing pain and discomfort.
- Promoting better structural and postural alignment.
- Enhancing circulation throughout your body.
- Improving your ability to exercise comfortably.
- Maintaining an overall healthy and enjoyable pregnancy.

The American College of Sport Medicine (ACSM), in the context of working with pregnant athletes, states *"professionals should strive to optimize alignment, muscle length tension and strength relationships, as well as muscle firing and movement during pregnancy."* This statement further reinforces the importance of maintaining a healthy spine and pelvis during pregnancy to minimize the impact of the musculoskeletal changes to your body.

Supporting You During the Postpartum Period
Following the birth of your child, these same practitioners can play a significant role in helping your body find its "new normal", coping with the physical demands of your training, and easing any muscle tension that you might experience as a result of breastfeeding and carrying your

newborn. As mentioned earlier, our bodies do not simply bounce back quickly after pregnancy and childbirth. If you are motivated to return to training sooner-rather-than-later, there can be serious consequences if you start to exercise more frequently and at a higher intensity before your body has properly healed. Involving certain practitioners in the postpartum phase may potentially help by:

- Speeding up your recovery from childbirth.
- Ensuring a healthy spine and pelvis.
- Correcting or reducing muscle tension.
- Improving function and correcting muscular weakness.
- Reducing your risk of injuries as you resume training.

Remember, some of the signs and symptoms that may occur during and after pregnancy might be subtle and go unnoticed initially. However, as time goes by, they could cause issues and perhaps pain. If addressed early on with a trained eye, the chance of them exploding into something more serious can be prevented.

General Considerations When Choosing a Practitioner

It can be difficult, even overwhelming at times, to decide which practitioner to see - especially given the different types of therapies and specialties available today. This decision is hard enough for you as an athlete, let alone a pregnant one! Part of the confusion may come from the overlap of the services offered by practitioners, as different practitioners can treat the same injuries or conditions successfully. In many cases, it is not just the type of practitioner that is important, but also their experience, philosophy and approach. This begs the question, *"How does one make a decision regarding which practitioner to see and when?"*

Although we will provide specific information regarding 5 different CAM professions that you may incorporate as part of your support team during and after your pregnancy, they are not the only CAM practitioners available. Therefore, it is important to consider the following when choosing a practitioner:

1. First and foremost, find someone experienced working with pregnant women. Such practitioners will likely have received additional training and will know how to address specific

pregnancy needs. Some techniques may need to be modified for your comfort and safety as your pregnancy progresses.

2. If you cannot find a practitioner that has experience working with pregnant women, choose someone who has worked with you in the past and is already familiar with your body and any past injuries. This will help them to assess the extent to which your body is changing and how these changes may impact you day-to-day.

3. If you have not already worked with a particular type of practitioner, ask a friend for a recommendation. Ideally, you would ask a friend you trust and preferably, someone who has been in a similar situation to you (i.e. pregnant and active).

4. Do not get discouraged. If the practitioner or the alternative therapy you choose is not working for you, try someone else or try a different therapy. It may not be the practitioner's skill level that is the problem; you may find that their personality or philosophy simply does not mesh with yours. That is ok! Just make sure you take the time to find the right person for you.

Although research in these particular areas may be limited, many practitioners have successfully treated women during and after their pregnancy for a variety of conditions. As always, it is recommended that you inform your primary health care provider of any additional care that you receive.

Exploring Different Types of Practitioners
It would be very easy to devote an entire book to this topic. To keep the information manageable (and to avoid confusing you), we have narrowed our focus to the following 5 types of practitioners, due to their popularity among athletes and the services that they can provide before, during and after your pregnancy:

- Physiotherapists
- Chiropractic doctors
- Registered massage therapists
- Osteopathic practitioners
- Naturopaths

This is not to say that other types of practitioners are of any less value. In fact, we encourage you to explore and consider any other profession that can be of assistance, especially if you have been working with them prior to getting pregnant. Just be diligent in your research and when in doubt, err on the side of caution.

Physiotherapists

As an athlete, you likely received treatment from a physiotherapist at some point in time. This is not surprising, as a large part of the physiotherapist's profession is to manage and prevent physical problems caused by sports-related injuries. However, they do a lot more than that. According to the Canadian Physiotherapy Association, physiotherapists manage and prevent many physical problems caused by illness, disease, sport and work-related injury, aging and long periods of inactivity. They are skilled in the assessment and management of a broad range of conditions that can affect the musculoskeletal, circulatory, respiratory and nervous systems.

A Rare but Valuable Resource

Physiotherapists are one of the few practitioners that may have pursued additional training to help you strengthen your pelvic floor muscles and make sure that you are doing the exercises correctly. This type of service can be extremely valuable during and after your pregnancy, as described in the chapter "Your Silent Training Partner – Your Pelvic Floor Muscles". A physiotherapist can also assist in finding a lower lumbar support belt, which may help to relieve discomfort in your lower back, especially while running or walking.

Given that most women will experience some form of musculoskeletal discomfort during/after their pregnancy, there are many ways in which a physiotherapist can continue to be involved in your care. Some of the more common pregnancy-related conditions that a physiotherapist may treat include:

- Lower back and pelvic pain caused by a shift in your centre of gravity during your pregnancy.
- Neck pain and headaches due to postural changes throughout your pregnancy and into the postpartum period.
- Tightness and pain in the hamstrings and heels as a result of mechanical changes in the feet (flattening of the arches).

- Bladder leakage during pregnancy and after delivery due to strained pelvic muscles.
- Weak pelvic floor muscles, with or without organ prolapse.
- Burning or tingling in the wrist as a result of weight and water gain (also known as carpal tunnel syndrome).
- Symphysis pubis separation (also known as pubic pain or pelvic girdle pain).

After your delivery, a physiotherapist may also be able to facilitate your return to an active lifestyle. Not only can they check for things like muscle imbalances or weaknesses, but they can also provide you with the proper exercises to help initiate your training.

Chiropractic Doctors

Although you may or may not have received care in the past from a chiropractor, these practitioners can also assist you in many ways. According the Canadian Chiropractic Association, their scope of practice consists of the examination, assessment, diagnosis, treatment, management and prevention of spinal, joint and related neuromuscular disorders. Chiropractors are specialists in spinal manipulation (also known as an "adjustment" or "crack") on the vertebrae of the spine and other joints of

> **Did You Hear That Pop?**
> Why do my joints pop when I get an adjustment? A chiropractic adjustment may result in release of a gas bubble between the joints – "the pop" – which is caused by the change of pressure within the joints. Rest assured that this is not necessarily painful and should not cause any harm.

the body where there may be a decreased movement in the joints. These adjustments may help reduce pain and restore normal function to the joints, supporting muscles and ligaments so you can get back to what you enjoy.

According to a recent study by Yuen et al. (2013), the most common types of treatment that chiropractors provided to pregnant women were patient education, soft tissue therapy, exercise therapies and spinal manipulative therapy. Despite the concerns or assumptions that people may have regarding chiropractic care (such as spinal manipulation), it is safe to see a chiropractor during your pregnancy. In fact, in a recent review of the literature, Stuber and colleagues (2012) found that problems following spinal manipulation were rare during pregnancy and postpartum. Furthermore, the American Pregnancy Association states that there are no known contraindications to chiropractic care throughout pregnancy, as chiropractors can provide safe, effective and drug-free conservative care. More specifically, a chiropractor may be involved during/after your pregnancy in the following ways:

- Providing spinal manipulation or adjustment at different points along your spine, including neck, upper and lower back or other joints of the body to promote optimal movement of those joints.
- Applying soft tissue therapies, such as Graston Technique and Active Release Technique (ART), to help decrease muscle tightness.
- Educating and encouraging posture correction throughout pregnancy and beyond, thereby stretching tight muscles and strengthening any muscle imbalances.
- Establishing balance in your pelvis and minimizing stress to the uterus and supporting ligaments. Chiropractors with additional training may apply a specific adjustment called "the Webster Technique" to achieve such balance.

Postpartum, a chiropractor can help you recover from the stresses of childbirth including pain, exhaustion and incontinence, by restoring proper mobility and assisting your natural healing process. Most chiropractors are also well versed in exercise therapy and can help you back to the road of physical activity.

Registered Massage Therapists
Many athletes welcome a nice massage during their training season. But did you know that massage therapy, a hands-on manipulation of the soft tissues of the body, including muscles, connective tissue, tendons, ligaments and joints, can do a lot more than alleviate sore muscles and discomfort?

Although there is only a small amount of research concerning massage therapy and pregnancy, the evidence suggests that prenatal massage may be beneficial. For instance, Field and colleagues (1999) demonstrated a significantly decreased intensity of pregnancy-related back pain, reduced anxiety, improved mood and better sleep following 22-minute massage therapy sessions 2 times per week in the 3rd trimester. In an earlier study, Field et al. (1997) found that massage during labour reduced the length of labour and time spent in the hospital, as well as lessened postpartum depression. Other studies found improved maternal mood, decreased pain and anxiety, decreased stress hormones, decreased obstetrical complications and improved neonatal health and development as a result of massage therapy. During and after your pregnancy, a registered massage therapist can help with:

- Improving the circulation of your blood and reducing any swelling.
- Decreasing the discomfort of varicose veins and hemorrhoids.
- Lessening any muscular pain and tension that you might be experiencing.
- Providing you with a sense of relaxation and well-being by reducing stress and anxiety.

Proper positioning during a massage will maximize your comfort level and avoid placing unnecessary pressure on your abdomen. Lying on your back for a short duration of time is usually fine early in your pregnancy, as long as you are comfortable and not feeling dizzy. Side-lying is another alternative, as this position can help to minimize any pressure to the abdomen or stretching of the uterine ligaments. Alternatively, you can try lying face down, as long as you use the proper supports to avoid placing pressure on your belly. This can be done with pillows or with the use of a special pregnancy massage pillow that has a hole cut out in the centre. It is important to discuss the various positions with your registered massage therapist and communicate any discomfort.

> **My Story: Taking Care of Myself**
> I was accustomed to frequent massages during peak training season. But these were not what I would consider "relaxing" massages. In fact, these deep tissue massages were usually quite painful and the relaxation came only once the massage was over. During my pregnancy, however, I treated myself to more relaxing and gentler massages. I continued to benefit from the muscle tension release, but more so from the sense of relaxation that came about during the massage. This was just one way that I could take better care of myself and my baby.
> *Jennifer Faraone, co-author, competitive duathlete and runner, mother of 2*

Although different types of massage therapy can be applied, the Swedish massage is popular among pregnant women as it addresses many common discomforts associated with pregnancy. A properly trained registered massage therapist will be aware of the pressure points on the wrist and ankles that should be avoided or applied with less pressure, as they can stimulate the uterus and potentially induce labour.

Osteopathic Practitioners

Although athletes seeking osteopathic care may not be as common as the previous 3 types of practitioners, this form of treatment is gaining popularity. Osteopathy views the human body as one complete unit made up of a large number of structures (e.g. organs and bones), systems (e.g. cardiovascular, hormonal) and functions that are interrelated. When a problem occurs in any of these 3 areas, signs and symptoms may appear elsewhere in the body. According to the Ontario Association of Osteopathic Manual Practitioners, a goal of osteopathy is to "maintain, improve or restore the normal physiological function of interrelated body structures and systems, and enhance the body's natural ability to health itself." One of the most noticeable differences between the treatments received from an osteopath practitioner, compared to the other practitioners, is the light touch or gentle techniques (including soft-tissue manipulation) used to release physical strain, restore normal body mechanics and re-establish balance among the body's systems. In most instances, you will not notice any pressure during the course of treatment. During your pregnancy, an osteopath practitioner can help your body adapt to its changes by focusing on:

- Enhancing structural alignment and mobility in the back, spine, pelvis and other joints.
- Improving circulation to address conditions such as swelling, varicose veins and hemorrhoids.
- Balancing the hormonal and nervous systems.
- Alleviating some of the other common discomforts of pregnancy, including indigestion and breathing difficulties.

Despite being practiced since the 1800's, there has been very limited research on the topic of osteopathy and pregnancy. However, this is slowly changing in response to the increased interest in osteopathy as a whole. For example, Licciardone and colleagues (2010) examined a group of pregnant women experiencing back pain in their 3rd trimester. They found that osteopathic manipulation slows or halts the deterioration of back pain in late pregnancy and suggest that osteopathic treatment be used as a complement to a pregnant woman's usual obstetric care.

It has also been suggested that osteopathic treatment not be limited to musculoskeletal issues. For instance, osteopathic practitioners can help to better position the baby and prepare the body for easier labour and delivery; this can be done by restoring balance and improving the quality of movements of the whole pelvic girdle through stretching, articulation and soft tissue techniques. Lavelle (2013), in his review of osteopathy as a treatment for pregnant women, reported that some of the earliest studies demonstrated a decrease in the average labour time in first time moms who received prenatal osteopathy treatment (9 hours and 54 minutes) versus those who did not (21 hours and 6 minutes). Such results are encouraging but it should be noted that additional research is required to confirm these earlier studies.

Following the birth of your child, an osteopath practitioner can also help to restore your body's balance and alleviate pain and discomfort that you might experience as a new mom. Treatments may include helping the organs, especially the uterus, bladder and intestines, return to their normal position and function.

Osteopathic Treatment During Pregnancy and Its Effect on Labour

Janet Walker, a registered osteopath and massage therapist, conducted a study involving 58 pregnant women (2007). A primary goal of the study was to determine the efficacy of monthly osteopathic treatments (starting in the 2nd trimester) on the outcomes of labour and delivery. She found that the average number of medical interventions decreased in those women who received treatment; specifically, epidurals and inductions were at significantly lower rates than those who did not receive treatment.

Naturopaths

More people than ever before are seeking and benefiting from naturopathic care. According to the Canadian Association of Naturopathic Doctors, naturopathic medicine blends modern scientific knowledge with traditional and natural forms of medicine. The focus is on balancing the mind, body and environment to achieve optimal health while supporting the body's natural ability to heal itself. Christine Matheson, a naturopath at Mahaya Forest Hill Integrative Health and MedCan Clinic, who has a special interest in women's health, explains that naturopathic medicine is part of a greater integrative or holistic health care plan. Working toward optimal health, patients can benefit from getting the best of both conventional medicine and complementary medicine.

Naturopathic treatments can include a range of natural medicine modalities that are tailored to the individual's physical and emotional needs. Such modalities may include clinical nutrition, botanical medicine, homeopathic medicine, traditional Chinese medicine (including herbal medicine and acupuncture), physical therapies and lifestyle counselling. During your pregnancy, you may benefit from naturopathic medicine in the following ways:

- Assessing the various factors that may be affecting your fertility, such as nutrition, stress, hormonal imbalance and overtraining.
- Creating a nutritional and vitamin/herbal supplement plan to optimize your health during your pregnancy.
- Managing some common pregnancy discomforts and concerns such as morning sickness, anemia, heartburn, constipation, emotional changes and vaginal yeast infections.
- Preparing your body for labour. Examples include providing herbal medicine to tone your uterus, creating a natural remedy kit for labour and providing recommendations to maximize your nutrition.
- Offering care postpartum to both you and your baby such as assisting with a successful breastfeeding experience, discussing the importance of Vitamin D and probiotic supplements for your newborn, facilitating your physical recovery as well as addressing any emotional concerns that may arise.

> **Specialized Care for the Athlete and Her Baby**
>
> As a pregnant athlete, you may see a naturopath for sport-related issues such as nutrition and injuries during your pregnancy. Christine Matheson from Mahaya Forest Hill Integrative Health and MedCan Clinic believes that proper nutrition, rest, exercise and stress management are fundamental for the pregnant athlete. Matheson focuses on prioritizing these 4 elements and, as necessary, will recommend natural supplements and herbs. "I believe that a more pure and simple approach is often best during pregnancy. I prefer to focus on natural lifestyle modifications, rather than overprescribing supplements, in order to allow nature to take its course," explains Matheson.

Summary

In addition to your obstetrician or midwife, your pregnancy support team may include other practitioners and can be a wonderful adjunct to your prenatal and postnatal care. Such practitioners may include, but are not limited to, physiotherapists, chiropractors, registered massage therapists, osteopathic practitioners and naturopaths. Together, they can potentially help manage many of the discomforts and pain associated with pregnancy, improve your labour experience and give your postpartum recovery a boost. When looking for a new practitioner, do not be afraid to ask around for referrals and be sure to ask them upfront about their experience working with pregnant women.

Chapter 20

YOUR STRONG AND POWERFUL CORE

My core is made up of which muscles?
Why is core strength so important during pregnancy?
Isn't it enough that I had toned abs before getting pregnant?

At the Core of It All

Your core consists of a group of muscles that act as a powerhouse to provide the necessary support, stability, strength and balance for your day-to-day activities, as well as your athletic endeavours. Although such reasons continue to be important now that you are pregnant (and hopefully active), there are some additional reasons why a strong core during your pregnancy and the postpartum period is essential (Table 20.0).

If you haven't already guessed it by now, a strong core is not simply about having a flat stomach and involves more than just your abdominal muscles; it also includes those of the hip, back, buttock and pelvic floor muscles, as mentioned previously in the chapter "Getting Yourself to the Start Line". That's a lot of muscles working together! With the role that they play in your day-to-day activities and athletic pursuits, it's no wonder that "core strength" is getting so much attention these days. It is for this reason we want to provide you with a basic overview of the core's anatomy, before jumping into a strengthening program that is tailored to the pregnant athlete.

Table 20.0: Role of Your Core Before, During and After Pregnancy

Why Your Core is Important	
Before	• Plays a central role when engaging in day-to-day activities such as working, taking care of children, sitting at your desk, etc. • Essential for improved performance in your sport or preferred activity. • Helps to prevent injuries including low back pain and hip or knee issues.
During	• Provides the necessary support to your body as your belly gets bigger. (e.g. a strong core helps to maintain proper posture). • Prevents pregnancy-related discomforts such as low back pain or pelvic girdle pain. • Helps you to remain active throughout your pregnancy. • Facilitates labour and may prevent tearing of the pelvic floor muscles and the need for an episiotomy. • Helps to prevents incontinence or organ prolapse.
After	• Lessens the risk of back pain that you may encounter as a result of the endless amount of bending over (e.g. when picking up your baby or baby gear, giving your child a bath or changing diapers). • Assists in day-to-day activities such as running after your little one as he or she becomes mobile. • Enables you to get back to your sport or preferred activity sooner, with less aches and pains. • Helps to prevent incontinence or organ prolapse.

A Tour of Your Core Muscles

While different sources may vary in their definition of what constitutes as the core, for the purpose of this chapter we will focus on the muscles from the following areas: your abdominals, back, buttock and hip. Each of these areas has their own set of muscles and below is a brief description of the ones that we are most concerned with. Your pelvic floor muscles, which are also considered part of your core, will be discussed in the next chapter "Your Silent Training Partner – Your Pelvic Floor Muscles".

Abdominal Muscles
There are 4 key abdominal muscles:

- **Rectus abdominis** - The most superficial of the 4 muscles, they run vertically up and down the front of your torso and are separated by a band of connective tissue known as the linea alba. You may know these as the "six-pack".
- **Internal/external obliques** – These 2 muscles are on either side of your torso. You may know these as the "love handles".
- **Transversus abdominis** - The deepest of all 4 muscles, they run lower down on the torso in a horizontal direction, like a corset. You may know these as the "lower abs".

Squeezing It Out...Toothpaste That Is!

Did you know that your abdominal muscles may facilitate the pushing part of your labour? Although you may only be thinking of "bearing down" with your pelvic floor muscles, ideally you should be using your transverse muscle as well, but in a different way. When pushing, you should be focusing on contracting your transverse muscles by pulling them in; at the same time, you should be relaxing your pelvic floor muscles. In her book Maternal Fitness, author Julie Tupler uses the analogy of squeezing toothpaste out of its tube. In order to get toothpaste out, you must squeeze at the top (squeezing your abdominal muscles) in order to get the toothpaste out. But if you do not relax the pelvic floor muscles, you are essentially leaving the cap on the tube. More information about how to practice squeezing your transverse muscle while opening up your pelvic floor muscles is provided in the chapter "Preparing For The Big Event".

Although your abdominal muscles work independently, they must also work together to achieve proper function and stability. These muscles function to move your spine in different directions such as when performing a crunch, bending over to pick something off the floor or twisting to hit a ball while playing baseball. Furthermore, your abdominal muscles work in tandem with your pelvic floor muscles during the pushing part of your labour. Training these 2 sets of muscles to work together will take some time and effort, but the pay-off could result in a more comfortable delivery. Refer to the chapter "Preparing For The Big Event" for more information on how to work your abdominal and pelvic floor muscles together.

Back Muscles

Your back muscles are comprised of multiple layers and within these layers are a number of muscles that work together to produce movement, ensuring stability and strength for your core. Rather than discussing each muscle individually, we will focus on those muscle groups that are closest to the spinal column. The most superficial of these are the erector spinae group – these are the long muscles that you can see on either side of your spine. Just under those and closer to the spine is a group of muscles known as the transversospinalis group. These 2 muscle groups run from your head to your tailbone and help to maintain your posture and control certain movements like extending and twisting the spine. Another muscle that plays a role in stabilizing the spine is the quadratus lumborum or quite simply, the QL. This thick, strong muscle is under the erector spinae muscles, running along the lower part of your spinal column on both sides and attaching to the pelvis. The role of the QL is to help stabilize the spine, flex or bend the spine sideways and elevate the hip.

Hip Muscles

Although commonly referred to as the "hip flexors", this area is actually comprised of 2 separate muscles - the psoas and the iliacus. These 2 muscles have different starting points that merge in the pelvis and then attach to the inside of your thigh. These muscles are an essential part of many movements such as walking and running, stabilizing the spine and flexing or bending your trunk.

Buttock Muscles

There are 4 buttock muscles - the gluteus maximus, gluteus medius, gluteus minimus and the tensor fascia lata. Generally, these muscles attach to your hip bones and to the outer part of your thighbone. The gluteus maximus is the largest and strongest of these muscles, helps to move your body and gives your backside (or your "booty") its shape. However, it is the other 3 muscles that work with the other muscles of the body to provide stability to your hips/pelvic region and spine.

Your Core's Transformation During Pregnancy

Your core muscles undergo a huge transformation during pregnancy. The most obvious change being your abdominal muscles, which stretches as your belly grows. At the same time, many of the muscles mentioned above are going through their own changes. As such, they affect not only each other, but may impact your body as a whole, often in the form of aches and pains. To further understand this concept, take into consideration the following research studies:

- Coldron and colleagues (2008) and Weis and colleagues (2009, 2011) have shown that the abdominal muscles change substantially during pregnancy, including the rectus abdominis and the internal oblique muscles that thins or stretches over the course of pregnancy. As your waistline increases, the rectus abdominis (and possibly the internal obliques) muscle will stretch and ultimately the linea alba may separate. When this happens, there may be reduced muscle activity, decreased stability and possibly pain in the low back and pelvis.
- Bewyer and colleagues (2009) found that pregnant women were between 6-8 times more likely to have low back pain if there was gluteus muscle weakness. The researchers suggested that this weakness, in conjunction with abdominal thinning, contributes to poor stabilization and back pain.
- Gutke and colleagues (2008) found that women who suffered from pelvic girdle pain (PGP) and/or combined pain (during and following pregnancy) had decreased erector spinae endurance and decreased hip strength during extension. The researchers suggested that this inadequacy may cause insufficient spinal stability (a decrease in the efficiency of how your body moves) combined with increased pain.

As demonstrated, such changes in the core muscles during pregnancy can cause a number of issues for the pregnant and postpartum body. These findings further reinforce the importance of a robust core training program before, during and following pregnancy. A program of this nature should be guided toward improving posture, increasing abdominal strength and improving lumbar/pelvic stability. In case you needed further convincing, consider the following: a recent systematic review of the literature by Van Benten et al. (2014) assessed the effectiveness of physical therapy (including exercise) in treating lumbar or pelvic pain during pregnancy. Nine studies in this review focused on exercise therapy and 7 studies focused on combined therapies such as exercise therapy and patient education. Almost all of these studies demonstrated that exercise helped to decrease pain and disability, improve function and/or limit sick leave for issues such as low back pain. Although the evidence for relieving PGP pain with exercise was still positive, it was a little less robust for this group. Furthermore, the author pointed out that the studies including individualized stabilization exercises appeared to be most beneficial to pregnant and postpartum women.

Working Your Core

After all this talk about the core and its complexity, you might be asking, "*how do you actually work the core, especially while pregnant*"? Here's the good news – it's probably easier than you think! First of all, if you were already accustomed to strengthening your core several times a week, there is a good chance that you can maintain most of your routine while pregnant with just a few exceptions. Second, working the core is more than performing an endless number of crunches; in fact, you may be surprised with many of the suggested exercises. For instance, many of the exercises

> **Stabilization is the Key!**
> "Stability" is achieved when your abdominal (and overall core) muscles work to maintain posture and balance while performing movement, thereby avoiding injury and pain. In non-pregnant studies McGill and colleagues (2007) developed the "Big 3" exercises to promote spinal stability including the modified curl up, side plank and bird dog. These exercises have been successful in alleviating injuries such as low back pain. Although a "Big 3" stability program for pregnant women does not currently exist, this topic is definitely gaining interest and new research is slowly starting to emerge. In fact, 2 recent case studies by Rajalakshmi and Kumar (2012) and Thein-Nissenbaum et al. (2012) demonstrated positive results in pregnant women who suffered from back pain by specifically training the transversus abdominis muscle.

will work your core while also challenging your sense of balance and proprioception (or knowing where your body/limbs are in terms of space). Both balance and proprioception are essential when it comes to performing your day-to-day activities, let alone exercising.

A Quick Check

Before starting these exercises, take a minute to check that you are doing the basic movement correctly. This is done quickly with an exercise known as "belly breathing" or "baby hugs", as it resembles giving your baby a hug from the inside.

- Lie on the floor, in the neutral spine position (i.e. make sure that there is space between the floor and your lower back).
- As you inhale and take a deep breath in, expand your stomach or "let it go". You should see your stomach getting bigger (yes, even bigger than what it already is!).
- As you exhale and breathe out, draw your belly button in as far as you can. Maintain the space between the floor and your lower back while exhaling. In other words, don't flatten your back.
- *Note:*
  - This is the movement/breathing that you want to incorporate with ALL of your core strength activities.
  - If this was difficult, you might want to practice this exercise several times until it feels natural to you, before moving on to the next set of exercises.

Should you start to feel dizzy or light headed while performing these exercises lying down, stop doing the activity and sit-up. This simply means that your body does not like being in that particular position for any period of time. Next time, try performing the exercises in the sitting or standing position.

Watch Those Curves!

Before engaging in any exercise, it is important to remember the following: there are 3 natural curves in your body: at the neck, the upper back and the lower back. This is known as your "neutral spine". Regardless of the exercise you perform, or whether it is done in standing, sitting or lying, it is important to maintain the curves in your body. If you are unsure what your neutral spine is, stand against a wall with your feet together, heels against the wall and feel the spaces between your back, neck and the wall - that is your neutral spine.

Suggested Exercises

Table 20.1 outlines several exercises that can help strengthen and stabilize your core while challenging your balance and proprioception. Two different sets of exercises are provided, based on your own level of strength, comfort and access to certain pieces of equipment, such as a BOSU, exercise ball or a rocker board. Alternatively, you can try performing some of the exercises while standing on one leg or with your eyes closed to make it more challenging. As with any type of exercise, the trick is to start off easy and then gradually make it more challenging. You can try several of these exercises in a session, completing 1-2 sets, aiming for 10-15 repetitions. Performing core strengthening exercises 2-3 times per week is ideal and a detailed description of each one is provided in Appendix 8.

Table 20.1: Suggested Core Strength Exercises

Initial	Progression
Baby Hugs (Belly Breathing)	Side Plank
Ball Curls	Plank
Single Leg ¼ Squat	Squats Off a BOSU
Monster Walk	Lunging On Top of a BOSU
Walking Lunge with Torso Twist	Bicep Curl Standing on One Foot
Hip Hikes	Shoulder Press Standing on a BOSU
Bridge	
Bird Dog	

Additional Considerations for Core Strengthening
Remember the following when doing any of the core strength exercises:

- ***Breathe.*** Avoid holding your breath during the exercises; ensure you are inhaling and exhaling.
- ***Curves are good.*** When doing these exercises, it is important to maintain the neutral curves in your lower back and neck.
- ***Variation is good.*** It is recommended to avoid exercises performed while lying on your back after your 4th month of pregnancy. If you want to continue with some of your previous exercises that had you lying on your back, try doing them in a semi-reclined position, such as on your exercise ball or on a semi-reclined workout bench.
- ***Separation is not good.*** If you have diastasis recti – a separation of your rectus abdominis muscles, it is important to avoid doing a large number of exercises that work your rectus and oblique (side) muscles, as this could lead to further separation of the muscles. Refer to the next section for more information.
- ***Seek help.*** If you are unsure of what to do, we encourage you to enlist the help of a qualified fitness or health care practitioner who understands how to strengthen your core during pregnancy.

Diastasis Recti

Diastasis recti (DR) is a condition where the connective tissue connecting the 2 halves of your abdominal muscles (more specifically the rectus abdominis) along the midline of your torso stretches and separates as a result of your growing belly. This separation can weaken the abdominal muscles and limit their functionality, not to mention leaving the lumbar spine and pelvis more prone to injury. DR also makes it impossible to regain a flat stomach.

DR can occur both during pregnancy and into the postpartum period, but occurs most frequently in the 3rd trimester. It has been stated that greater than 66% of pregnant women will suffer from this condition. Other studies have suggested that greater than 50% of women will experience DR in the postpartum period. Women are more susceptible to developing DR if they are pregnant over the age of 35, are carrying multiples (twins, triplets, etc.), have had more than one pregnancy or if they are carrying a larger child. According to some research, regular exercise prior to and during pregnancy may reduce the chance of getting DR and/or decrease the size of the separation.

DR is usually diagnosed when you have a separation that is greater than 2.7cm (approximately 2 fingertips) when measured at the belly button (or just above/below). It may be easier to see the separation, or the bulging along the midline of your belly, when performing a simple abdominal exercise. You can follow this simple procedure yourself to determine if you have DR (Figure 20.0):

- Lie on your back, knees bent with one hand behind your head and one hand at the level of the belly button.
- Slowly lift your head and shoulders off the ground as though you are going to do a crunch or curl up.
- Hold your head and shoulders off the ground for a few seconds and use your free hand to determine how many fingertips, if any, fit horizontally into the separation.

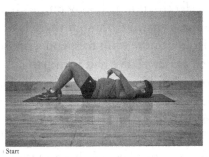
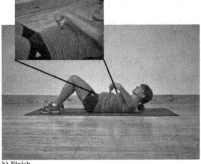

Start   b) Finish

Figure 20.0: Diastasis Recti

Strengthening your core is important if you have DR; however, some modifications are required:

- From the research presented so far, stabilization exercises are key. Consider starting with belly breathing or baby hugs, modified plank and bird dog (refer to Appendix 8).
- Until your separation is minimized, it is best to avoid exercises that specifically contract your oblique (side) or rectus abdominis muscles, such as side-to-side or regular crunches. These exercises could lead to further separation of the stomach muscles. This does not mean that you will never be able to perform a crunch ever again. You just want to make sure that your body is ready for that particular exercise.
- When you start incorporating crunches (side to side or regular), you should try the following technique: prior to getting into the crunch position, wrap a scarf, shawl, or towel behind your lower back, and hold an end in each hand. Then, cross each end over your stomach and gently pull each side toward the midline of your body. This should feel snug and will help to keep your muscles together while doing your crunch. Don't have a scarf or towel? You can provide the same type of support by simply crossing your arms over your stomach and gently pulling the muscles inward.
- Seek help from a qualified exercise or health care practitioner that has experience with DR. They can ensure that you are doing the correct exercise in the appropriate manner. Otherwise, you risk worsening the separation.

Your Beautiful Belly

Think that we are referring to the perfectly rounded baby bump that you showcased during pregnancy? Guess again! Although there is no doubt that a pregnant belly is beautiful, we now want to spend a bit of time talking about your beautiful belly after you've had your baby. As is the case for many women, your stomach following childbirth may be a "taboo" part of your body; it can be easy to focus on the excess weight and the loss of muscle definition in this area. But that doesn't mean your core muscles are non-existent! Although they may be in hiding and may be weak, these muscles are important in re-establishing support, strength and stability. So rather than focusing on what it looks like on the outside, try to appreciate your core for what it is doing on the inside. Remember that there is a very good reason why your stomach looks the way it does after childbirth – it went through many changes to create the nurturing environment for your growing baby. And that is really a beautiful thing!

Strengthening your core may seem daunting at first, especially if you are feeling emotionally and physically exhausted following the birth of your baby. As with many new moms, you are probably taking care of everyone else and before you know it, time has passed and you have not done anything for yourself. Carving out time to eat properly and exercise can be challenging, leading to frustration with the lack of progress toward your fitness goals, weight loss and the dreaded "mummy tummy" or "baby bulge". The good news is that you can take matters into your own hands and tackle that dreaded area. The even better news is that you don't need to wait until you are able to commit to a full-blown training program; you can start to see improvement in your core with only a few simple exercises each day. These exercises can be done in 5-10 minutes in the comfort of your home, with your newborn nearby.

You can likely start to strengthen your core shortly following the birth of your child, once you are feeling up to it. A good place to start is with belly breathing or baby hugs, as described earlier. After that, you can proceed with body-weighted core activities, prior to moving onto those activities that require equipment. This approach may also be more convenient if you are spending additional time at home in the first few months following the birth of your child. We suggest starting with the following core exercises (Appendix 8):

- Belly breathing
- Ball curl
- Side plank
- Plank
- Bird dog

At the same time, it is a good idea to perform your pelvic floor strengthening exercises, starting with the basic contractions as described in the chapter "Your Silent Training Partner – Your Pelvic Floor Muscles". As you feel ready, you can slowly begin to add in 1 or 2 exercises and see how your body responds. If you have any questions or uncertainties about starting a strengthening program for your core, speak to your health care provider at your postpartum check-up or see one of the other health care or exercise professionals we have discussed previously. Additional time will be required if you had a caesarean section, as your body will require more time to heal. Although you may be able to perform the baby hugs (belly breathing) and the pelvic floor exercises right way, you should wait until your postpartum check-up before starting the other exercises.

Summary
A strong core before, during and following pregnancy is essential. In fact, a strong core can help to minimize pain and discomfort, provide better support in your daily activities and exercises and can even facilitate labour. Devoting just a little bit of time each day to perform the suggested exercises will go a long way toward helping you during your pregnancy, as well as facilitating your comeback to your sport afterward.

Chapter 21

YOUR SILENT TRAINING PARTNER – YOUR PELVIC FLOOR MUSCLES

Why should I be paying attention to my pelvic floor muscles?
Isn't it just older people that need to worry about them?
Can I still exercise if I have weak pelvic floor muscles, incontinence or a prolapse?

Why the Hype?

Let's face it - most women do not spend a lot of time thinking about their pelvic floor muscles. Many women probably have the perception that it is only the elderly who suffer from leaky bladders and who have to worry about these muscles. But that is far from the truth! Pelvic floor weakness (and its related conditions) is more common than you think and affects younger women as well, often starting during the pregnancy and postpartum periods. It has even been suggested that the stress of childbirth on the pelvic floor muscles can last for almost a decade! Other sources have reported the following:

- Nygaard (1997) found that nearly 36% of female Olympians who participated in high impact sports were more likely to report urinary incontinence in comparison to low level impact activity athletes.
- A later study by Nygaard and colleagues (2008) reported that simply being a woman gives you a 13% chance of pelvic floor dysfunction. This risk increases to 18% following the birth of your first child, then to a whopping 32% if you had 3 babies.

- A study by Williams and colleagues (2007) found that 87% of women reported some type of perineum problem a year after giving birth; this included women who did not have any tears or an episiotomy during labour.

Oops, I Peed My Pants!
Incontinence, defined as the inability to control your urination, can be a common and embarrassing problem. It affects people of all ages and genders; however, it is more common among women, with pregnancy and vaginal delivery being risk factors. The symptoms and severity of urinary incontinence ranges from occasionally leaking urine when coughing or sneezing, to having an urge to urinate that's so sudden and strong you don't get to a toilet in time. The different types of urinary incontinence include:

- *Stress Incontinence:* Involuntary urine leakage prompted by a physical movement or activity (e.g. coughing, sneezing, running or heavy lifting) that puts pressure on your bladder. This is more common during and after pregnancy.
- *Urge Incontinence:* Involuntary urine leakage associated with, or immediately following, a sudden need to urinate. This form of incontinence is sometimes referred to as an overactive bladder.
- *Mixed Incontinence:* A combination of stress and urgency urinary incontinence.

In addition to urinary incontinence, some women also experience fecal or bowel incontinence, which is the inability to control your bowel movements. Some women may experience this after pregnancy if the anal sphincters or their nerves were affected during childbirth.

No wonder we have devoted an entire chapter on your pelvic floor muscles. While they form the base of the muscles typically referred to as your "core", the pelvic floor muscles are considered the "black sheep" of the core family. They are often neglected and seldom talked about unless there is a problem. Although you may not realize it, your pelvic floor muscles serve several important functions including:

- Supporting your organs in place (i.e. uterus, bladder and bowels).
- Supporting sphincter control of the bladder and bowels and organ prolapse.
- Enhancing sexual enjoyment.
- Supporting your baby during pregnancy and facilitating the birth process.

And contrary to what you might think, it is not just the weakness of these muscles that can be problematic. In fact, the inability to fully *relax* the muscles, as opposed to contracting them, can also have implications for your labour. Consider for a moment the muscles surrounding your vagina that must stretch to allow for your baby's head to emerge. If these muscles are too tight and not able to fully relax, an episiotomy may be required to prevent the tearing of these muscles.

So, should you be concerned with relaxing or strengthening these muscles? The answer is "yes" to both. Being able to fully relax the muscles is important for the reason mentioned above - to facilitate childbirth. On the other hand, it is important to promote or maintain adequate strength of these muscles during and after your pregnancy. Some of the pregnancy-related changes that your body experiences, including the weight of your baby on your pelvic floor, can weaken and add further stress on these muscles. So perhaps the focus should be on having "healthy" pelvic floor muscles, to characterize the need for both strengthening and relaxing.

What's Going on Down There?

Something just doesn't feel right down there? Do you suspect that you might have a prolapse? A prolapse literally means "to fall out of place" and there are 3 different types:

- *Uterine prolapse* - The cervix and uterus move down into the vagina.
- *Bladder prolapse (cystocoele)* - A downward movement of the bladder into the front wall of the vagina.
- *Bowel prolapse (rectocele)* – Part of the bowel, close to the rectum, moves down into the back wall of the vagina.

Although the symptoms may vary from woman to woman and depend on the type of prolapse, you may experience any of the following:

- Sensation of a bulge or a "lump" in the vagina
- Heavy feeling or "pulling down" in the vagina area
- Visible bulge from the vagina
- Difficulty inserting or retaining tampons
- Incontinence or difficulty emptying your bowels properly

If you suspect that you might have a prolapse, see your doctor and seek help from a qualified professional.

Pelvic Floor Anatomy 101

What are your pelvic floor muscles? In general, these are the layers of muscles that support the pelvic organs such as your bladder, bowel and uterus. These muscles form a sling that attaches to your tailbone and pubic bone and act as a hammock to support your pelvic organs (Figure 21.0).

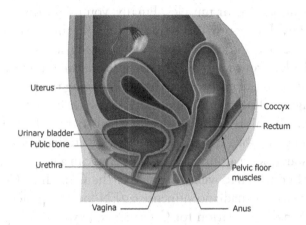

Uterus

Coccyx

Rectum

Urinary bladder
Pubic bone

Urethra

Pelvic floor
muscles

Vagina

Anus

Figure 21.0: Your Pelvic Floor

Learning how to activate your pelvic floor muscles can be a bit tricky, especially if you have not done it before. In fact, 1/3 of women squeeze the wrong muscles when trying to do a pelvic floor contraction, also known as a "Kegel" exercise; often it is the abdominal or buttock muscles that are contracted and not the pelvic floor muscles. By definition, a pelvic floor contraction is an inward lift and squeeze by the muscles of the pelvic floor. The easiest way to locate the pelvic floor muscles is as follows: the next time you are urinating, try focusing on your using your pelvic floor muscles to stop the flow of urine for 5-10 seconds. Feel which muscles are being used to stop the flow - these are your pelvic floor muscles. It is important that you do not practice this movement too often while urinating, as it could lead to a urinary tract infection.

Now, try squeezing the pelvic floor muscles while you are not urinating and see if you can mimic the same movement. You can also try this movement in various positions such as lying, sitting or standing. Remember to keep the muscles of the abdomen and buttocks (including the anus) relaxed.

Still having trouble locating these muscles and performing a contraction? Your partner may be able to help. During intercourse, stop for a moment and try to squeeze your partner's penis or fingers. If your partner can feel the contraction, then you are indeed activating the correct muscles; if not, keep working at it, as practice makes perfect! Alternatively, there are several pelvic floor devices that can help to strengthen the pelvic floor muscles and/or provide immediate feedback on the activation of your muscles. Finally, you might find it useful to speak to a health care provider who is trained in this area. Just as you would ask a coach to help perfect your running stride or a personal trainer to look at your form during strength training, there are trained professionals who can ensure that you are engaging the proper muscles.

Although finding such a professional may have been difficult in the past, fortunately, this is a growing field in which more and more resources are becoming available. If you are not aware of a trained professional in your area, start asking around for referrals. You can also check your local or national continence website, such as the Canadian Continence Foundation (www.canadiancontinence.ca/EN/locate-a-professional.php) or the National Association for Continence (www.nafc.org/find-an-expert), as they can help locate trained professionals in your area. In general, these professionals can:

- Assess your pelvic floor muscles and determine appropriate treatment approach.
- Teach you how to perform the strengthening exercises correctly (including how to isolate those muscles).
- Release muscle tension or treat scar tissue of the muscles.
- Treat incontinence and prolapse.
- Use additional forms of treatment, including biofeedback, muscle stimulation or vaginal weights, as required.

A Potential Training Partner?

Wouldn't it be great to have a tool that promotes pelvic floor wellness and can be used in the privacy of your home? There is! Different products are available ranging from weights to biofeedback and electrical stimulation devices. For instance, a vaginal cone is a weighted device that inserts into the vagina to make your strengthening exercises more challenging by isolating the appropriate muscles and giving you something to focus on. In addition, biofeedback and electrical stimulation devices provide positive reinforcement by helping you find the correct muscle group. Some devices come equipped with a pressure display (similar to what you would see on a blood pressure cuff) to provide immediate biofeedback on the strength and endurance of your pelvic floor muscles. Finally, some products can assist with stretching your perineum prior to your delivery in an effort to reduce the likelihood of tearing and strengthening your pelvic floor following delivery.

- Provide additional tips and suggestions regarding behavioural changes, such as diet and liquid intake, bladder retraining, exercise, etc.

Work Those Muscles

Although it can be a little disheartening to know just how common pelvic floor muscle weakness or its related conditions can be, the good news is that these muscles are very responsive to strengthening exercises or rehabilitation. In fact, an extensive review by Dumoulin and Hay-Smith (2010) demonstrated encouraging results of the effects of pelvic floor muscle training (PFMT) on incontinence before, during and after pregnancy. For example:

- Women with stress incontinence were up to 17 times more likely to notice improvement in their symptoms with PFMT.
- Women who participated in PFMT were approximately 50% less likely to experience incontinence shortly after giving birth.
- Women treated with PFMT were more likely to report cure or improvement, better quality of life, fewer leakage episodes and less urine leakage.

But you don't need to wait until you experience weakness before starting to strengthen these muscles. You can even begin *before* your pregnancy. Remember, the stronger these muscles are now, the stronger and better equipped the pelvic floor muscles will be to take on the demands of pregnancy. Jessica Zelinka, a Canadian Olympic heptathlete, 100m hurdler and mother of 1, knew the importance of maintaining strong pelvic floor muscles and was proactive about seeing a physiotherapist early on. Several years after the birth of her daughter, she continues to incorporate the exercises into her daily routine and encourages other women to do the same.

One More Reason

Female athletes participating in weight-bearing sports are at greater risk of urinary incontinence. Many researchers including Bo and Backe-Hansen (2007) suggest that athletes wanting to continue high level competitive sports consider strategies such as pelvic floor strengthening exercises to prevent or minimize these risks. Maybe it's time to start flexing those muscles!

Your pelvic floor muscles should not only be strong, but they should also be "fast" and resistant to fatigue. Therefore, a comprehensive PFMT program should include the basic contraction (or Kegel) exercise and some variation to incorporate strength, endurance, coordination and speed of the contraction. If this sounds a bit intimidating, relax. Training these muscles is just like training any other muscle where you start off easy and progress to a more challenging level. Assuming that you were successful in isolating and contracting your pelvic floor muscles (as described above), begin with the following routine:

Basic Contractions
- Lie down, with your knees bent and feet firmly planted on the floor. Perform a contraction and hold for several seconds. You may only be able to hold the contraction for 1-2 seconds but eventually you should work your way to 5-10 seconds.
- Relax the muscles for a few seconds. You have just completed 1 repetition.
- Aim to complete 8-12 repetitions in a row, making 1 set. After a short break, try repeating for 1 or 2 more sets.
- Perform the pelvic floor exercises in a controlled manner and avoid holding your breath.
- Aim to complete this exercise several times a day.
- Try executing the exercises in different positions, such as sitting and standing.

Once you have mastered the basic contraction, you can add some variations to your workout with the following exercises. Remember to keep breathing and avoid engaging your buttocks or abdominal muscles.

Elevator
Think of an elevator that goes up and down to different floors of an apartment building. You are going to control how high and how low your pelvic floor muscles are working by contracting and releasing them appropriately. For example, imagine there are 3 floors to your building. Draw the pelvic floor muscles up slowly to floor 1, then floor 2, then floor 3. Release the pelvic floor muscles completely as though you are going into the "basement".

As you start to gain more strength and control, you can try adding a few more floors to the elevator (e.g. going up to floor 5) or going back down a floor at a time (e.g. up 1-2-3-4-5 and down 4-3-2-1). You can also vary the movement by going up and down the floors in a non-linear fashion (e.g. 1-2-1-2-3-2-3-4-3-4). The idea is to keep some amount of muscle activation (contraction) while working on the coordination of the pelvic floor muscles. However, don't forget about going into the basement – you need to continue to teach your pelvic floor muscles to fully relax throughout this exercise (e.g. 1-2-1-2-3-4-2-3-4-basement).

Pulses (Quick Contractions)
Think of the following exercise as a series of mini pulses or short and quick movements. Perform the basic contraction but this time, try squeezing the muscles harder for a very brief moment and then quickly release. This is 1 repetition. Initiate the next repetition as soon as you feel that your muscles have relaxed. In other words, there is not much of a break between squeezes, and each one is small but powerful. Aim for 5-10 repetitions, provided that you can relax the muscles in between each contraction.

As mentioned earlier in this chapter, healthy pelvic floor muscles can facilitate the pushing part of your labour. Although you may not realize it, your abdominal muscles work closely with your pelvic floor muscles during the pushing part of labour. Training these muscles to work together during labour will take some time and effort, but the payoff could result in a more comfortable delivery. Refer to the chapter "Preparing Yourself For The Big Event" for more information on how to work your abdominal and pelvic floor muscles in tandem.

Modifying Your Workouts
If you experience incontinence or prolapse, you may be wondering if it is appropriate to exercise and whether certain forms of activities are more suitable than others. The good (and encouraging) news is that incontinence or prolapse does not necessarily mean that you must discontinue exercising. The truth of the matter is that there is no single exercise prescription for every woman; what it really comes down to is choosing a form of exercise that matches the ability of your pelvic floor muscles. Determining this ability is best done in consultation with an appropriate health care professional who can assess your pelvic floor function and provide appropriate recommendations.

What about weight-bearing activities such as running or jumping? Dragana Boljanovic-Susic, a registered physiotherapist with training in pelvic floor conditions, explains that there may be a number of factors that contribute to prolapse occurrence. Therefore the cause and progression can vary on a case-by-case basis and depends on the strength of your pelvic floor muscles, the extent of your prolapse, the intensity of your activity and your own comfort level. For example, if you have a minor pelvic organ prolapse and are strengthening your pelvic floor muscles on a daily basis, you may find that you can tolerate running without any increases in symptoms. On the other hand, if you notice an increase in symptoms either during or after the weight-bearing activity, it may be a sign that your pelvic floor muscles cannot provide adequate support for this particular workout. You might then need to modify the workout – either by scaling back the duration or switching to a lower impact activity. If you have a more significant prolapse, you may wish to consult an appropriate professional (i.e. OBGYN) to discuss additional treatment options such as a pessary (a device placed in your vagina to hold the prolapsed organ(s) in place) and in some cases, surgery.

> **The Unpleasant Side of Jumping**
> After the birth of my second child, I participated in local Cross Fit classes involving a lot of skipping and jumping up and down on a tall box. As you can imagine, both activities produced unappealing effects - and I wasn't the only one in the class with this issue. Let's just say that it was a good thing that I was wearing black tights! My symptoms of incontinence lasted for over a year.
> *Leslie Black, competitive runner, mother of 2*

Summary

After reading this chapter, we hope that you have a better understanding and appreciation as to why we call the pelvic floor muscles "your silent training partner". Although these muscles are often neglected, they play such an important role during and after pregnancy, as well as in your everyday life. If given a little bit of attention, they will support you; if neglected, they may not be there when they are needed most. Seeking help from a qualified professional can help to ensure that you are engaging these muscles properly while achieving pelvic floor wellness.

APPENDICES

APPENDICES

APPENDIX 1

PARmed-X for PREGNANCY

PHYSICAL ACTIVITY READINESS MEDI-
CAL EXAMINATION

PARmed-X for PREGNANCY is a guideline for health screening prior to participation in a prenatal fitness class or other exercise.

Healthy women with uncomplicated pregnancies can integrate physical activity into their daily living and can participate without significant risks either to themselves or to their unborn child. Postulated benefits of such programs include improved aerobic and muscular fitness, promotion of appropriate weight gain, and facilitation of labour. Regular exercise may also help to prevent gestational glucose intolerance and pregnancy-induced hypertension.

The safety of prenatal exercise programs depends on an adequate level of maternal-fetal physiological reserve. PARmed-X for PREGNANCY is a convenient checklist and prescription for use by health care providers to evaluate pregnant patients who want to enter a prenatal fitness program and for ongoing medical surveillance of exercising pregnant patients.

Instructions for use of the 4-page PARmed-X for PREGNANCY are the following:

1. The patient should fill out the section on PATIENT INFORMATION and the PRE-EXERCISE HEALTH CHECKLIST (PART 1, 2, 3, and 4 on p. 1) and give the form to the health care provider monitoring her pregnancy.
2. The health care provider should check the information provided by the patient for accuracy and fill out SECTION C on CONTRAINDICATIONS (p. 2) based on current medical information.
3. If no exercise contraindications exist, the HEALTH EVALUATION FORM (p. 3) should be completed, signed by the health care provider, and given by the patient to her prenatal fitness professional.

In addition to prudent medical care, participation in appropriate types, intensities and amounts of exercise is recommended to increase the likelihood of a beneficial pregnancy outcome. PARmed-X for PREGNANCY provides recommendations for individualized exercise prescription (p. 3) and program safety (p. 4).

NOTE: Sections A and B should be completed by the patient before the appointment with the health care provider.

A PATIENT INFORMATION

NAME

ADDRESS

TELEPHONE _____ BIRTHDATE _____ HEALTH INSURANCE No. _____

NAME OF
PRENATAL FITNESS PROFESSIONAL _____

PRENATAL FITNESS
PROFESSIONAL'S PHONE NUMBER _____

B PRE-EXERCISE HEALTH CHECKLIST

PART 1: GENERAL HEALTH STATUS

In the past, have you experienced (check YES or NO):

	YES	NO
1. Miscarriage in an earlier pregnacy?	❏	❏
2. Other pregnancy complications?	❏	❏
3. I have completed a PAR-Q within the last 30 days.	❏	❏

If you answered YES to question 1 or 2, please explain:

Number of previous pregnancies? _____

PART 2: STATUS OF CURRENT PREGNANCY

Due Date: _____

During this pregnancy, have you experienced:

	YES	NO
1. Marked fatigue?	❏	❏
2. Bleeding from the vagina ("spotting")?	❏	❏
3. Unexplained faintness or dizziness?	❏	❏
4. Unexplained abdominal pain?	❏	❏
5. Sudden swelling of ankles, hands or face?	❏	❏
6. Persistent headaches or problems with headaches?	❏	❏
7. Swelling, pain or redness in the calf of one leg?	❏	❏
8. Absence of fetal movement after 6th month?	❏	❏
9. Failure to gain weight after 5th month?	❏	❏

If you answered YES to any of the above questions, please explain:

PART 3: ACTIVITY HABITS DURING THE PAST MONTH

1. List only regular fitness/recreational activities:

INTENSITY	FREQUENCY (times/week)			TIME (minutes/day)		
	1-2	2-4	4+	<20	20-40	40+
Heavy	—	—	—	—	—	—
Medium	—	—	—	—	—	—
Light	—	—	—	—	—	—

2. Does your regular occupation (job/home) activity involve:

	YES	NO
Heavy Lifting?	❏	❏
Frequent walking/stair climbing?	❏	❏
Occasional walking (>once/hr)?	❏	❏
Prolonged standing?	❏	❏
Mainly sitting?	❏	❏
Normal daily activity?	❏	❏
3. Do you currently smoke tobacco?*	❏	❏
4. Do you consume alcohol?*	❏	❏

PART 4: PHYSICAL ACTIVITY INTENTIONS

What physical activity do you intend to do?

Is this a change from what you currently do?   ❏ YES   ❏ NO

*NOTE: PREGNANT WOMEN ARE STRONGLY ADVISED NOT TO SMOKE OR CONSUME ALCOHOL DURING PREGNANCY AND DURING LACTATION.

1

Physical Activity Readiness
Medical Examination for
Pregnancy

PARmed-X for PREGNANCY

PHYSICAL ACTIVITY READINESS MEDI-
CAL EXAMINATION

C CONTRAINDICATIONS TO EXERCISE: to be completed by your health care provider

Absolute Contraindications			Relative Contraindications		
Does the patient have:	YES	NO	*Does the patient have:*	YES	NO
1. Ruptured membranes, premature labour?	❏	❏	1. History of spontaneous abortion or premature labour in previous pregnancies?	❏	❏
2. Persistent second or third trimester bleeding/placenta previa?	❏	❏	2. Mild/moderate cardiovascular or respiratory disease (e.g., chronic hypertension, asthma)?	❏	❏
3. Pregnancy-induced hypertension or pre-eclampsia?	❏	❏	3. Anemia or iron deficiency? (Hb < 100 g/L)?	❏	❏
4. Incompetent cervix?	❏	❏	4. Malnutrition or eating disorder (anorexia, bulimia)?	❏	❏
5. Evidence of intrauterine growth restriction?	❏	❏	5. Twin pregnancy after 28th week?	❏	❏
6. High-order pregnancy (e.g., triplets)?	❏	❏	6. Other significant medical condition?	❏	❏
7. Uncontrolled Type I diabetes, hypertension or thyroid disease, other serious cardiovascular, respiratory or systemic disorder?	❏	❏	Please specify: _____		

NOTE: Risk may exceed benefits of regular physical activity. The decision to be physically active or not should be made with qualified medical advice.

PHYSICAL ACTIVITY RECOMMENDATION: ❏ Recommended/Approved ❏ Contraindicated

Prescription for Aerobic Activity

RATE OF PROGRESSION: The best time to progress is during the second trimester since risks and discomforts of pregnancy are lowest at that time. Aerobic exercise should be increased gradually during the second trimester from a minimum of 15 minutes per session, 3 times per week (at the appropriate target heart rate or RPE to a maximum of approximately 30 minutes per session, 4 times per week (at the appropriate target heart rate or RPE).

WARM-UP/COOL-DOWN: Aerobic activity should be preceded by a brief (10-15 min.) warm-up and followed by a short (10-15 min.) cool-down. Low intensity calesthenics, stretching and relaxation exercises should be included in the warm-up/cool-down.

PRESCRIPTION/MONITORING OF INTENSITY: The best way to prescribe and monitor exercise is by combining the heart rate and rating of perceived exertion (RPE) methods.

HEART RATE RANGES FOR PREGNANT WOMEN

MATERNAL AGE	FITNESS LEVEL or BMI	HEART RATE RANGE (beats/minute)
Less than 20	-	140-155
20–29	Low	129-144
	Active	135-150
	Fit	145-160
	BMI>25 kg m⁻²	102-124
30–39	Low	128-144
	Active	130-145
	Fit	140-156
	BMI>25 kg m⁻²	101-120

Target HR ranges were derived from peak exercise tests in medically prescreened low-risk women who were pregnant. (Mottola et al., 2006; Davenport et al., 2008).

RATING OF PERCEIVED EXERTION (RPE)

Check the accuracy of your heart rate target zone by comparing it to the scale below. A range of about 12-14 (somewhat hard) is appropriate for most pregnant women.

6	
7	Very, very light
8	
9	Somewhat light
10	
11	Fairly light
12	
13	Somewhat hard
14	
15	Hard
16	
17	Very hard
18	
19	Very, very hard
20	

F   **I**   **T**   **T**

FREQUENCY	INTENSITY	TIME	TYPE
Begin at 3 times per week and progress to four times per week	Exercise within an appropriate RPE range and/or target heart rate zone	Attempt 15 minutes, even if it means reducing the intensity. Rest intervals may be helpful	Non weight-bearing or low-impact endurance exercise using large muscle groups (e.g., walking, stationary cycling, swimming, aquatic exercises, low impact aerobics)

"TALK TEST" - A final check to avoid overexertion is to use the "talk test". The exercise intensity is excessive if you cannot carry on a verbal conversation while exercising.

The original PARmed-X for PREGNANCY was developed by L.A. Wolfe, Ph.D., Queen's University and updated by Dr. M.F. Mottola, Ph.D., University of Western Ontario.

No changes permitted. Translation and reproduction in its entirety is encouraged.

Disponible en français sous le titre «Examination medicale sur l'aptitude à l'activité physique pour les femmes enceintes (X-AAP pour les femmes enceintes)»

Additional copies of the PARmed-X for PREGNANCY, can be downloaded from

Canadian Society for Exercise Physiology
www.csep.ca/forms

2

Physical Activity Readiness
Medical Examination for
Pregnancy

PARmed-X for PREGNANCY

Prescription for Muscular Conditioning

It is important to condition all major muscle groups during both prenatal and postnatal periods.

WARM-UPS & COOL DOWN: *Range of Motion:* neck, shoulder girdle, back, arms, hips, knees, ankles, etc.

Static Stretching: all major muscle groups

(DO NOT OVER STRETCH!)

EXAMPLES OF MUSCULAR STRENGTHENING EXERCISES

CATEGORY	PURPOSE	EXAMPLE
Upper back	Promotion of good posture	Shoulder shrugs, shoulder blade pinch
Lower back	Promotion of good posture	Modified standing opposite leg & arm lifts
Abdomen	Promotion of good posture, prevent low-back pain, prevent diastasis recti, strengthen muscles of labour	Abdominal tightening, abdominal curl-ups, head raises lying on side or standing position
Pelvic floor ("Kegels")	Promotion of good bladder control, prevention of urinary incontinence	"Wave", "elevator"
Upper body	Improve muscular support for breasts	Shoulder rotations, modified push-ups against a wall
Buttocks, lower limbs	Facilitation of weight-bearing, prevention of varicose veins	Buttocks squeeze, standing leg lifts, heel raises

PRECAUTIONS FOR MUSCULAR CONDITIONING DURING PREGNANCY

VARIABLE	EFFECTS OF PREGNANCY	EXERCISE MODIFICATIONS
Body Position	• in the supine position (lying on the back), the enlarged uterus may either decrease the flow of blood returning from the lower half of the body as it presses on a major vein (inferior vena cava) or it may decrease flow to a major artery (abdominal aorta)	• past 4 months of gestation, exercises normally done in the supine position should be altered • such exercises should be done side lying or standing
Joint Laxity	• ligaments become relaxed due to increasing hormone levels • joints may be prone to injury	• avoid rapid changes in direction and bouncing during exercises • stretching should be performed with controlled movements
Abdominal Muscles	• presence of a rippling (bulging) of connective tissue along the midline of the pregnant abdomen (diastasis recti) may be seen during abdominal exercise	• abdominal exercises are not recommended if diastasis recti develops
Posture	• increasing weight of enlarged breasts and uterus may cause a forward shift in the centre of gravity and may increase the arch in the lower back • this may also cause shoulders to slump forward	• emphasis on correct posture and neutral pelvic alignment. Neutral pelvic alignment is found by bending the knees, feet shoulder width apart, and aligning the pelvis between accentuated lordosis and the posterior pelvic tilt position.
Precautions for Resistance Exercise	• emphasis must be placed on continuous breathing throughout exercise • exhale on exertion, inhale on relaxation using high repetitions and low weights • Valsalva Manoevre (holding breath while working against a resistance) causes a change in blood pressure and therefore should be avoided • avoid exercise in supine position past 4 months gestation	

✂ ....

PARmed-X for Pregnancy - Health Evaluation Form
(to be completed and given to the prenatal fitness professional after obtaining medical clearance to exercise)

I, _____ PLEASE PRINT (patient's name), have discussed my plans to participate in physical activity during my current pregnancy with my health care provider and I have obtained his/her approval to begin participation.

Signed: _____   Date: _____
      (patient's signature)

                                                  HEALTH CARE PROVIDER'S COMMENTS:

Name of health care provider: _____

Address: _____

_____

Telephone: _____

                                           (health care provider's signature)

3

© Canadian Society for Exercise Physiology, 2013

Jennifer Faraone & Dr. Carol Ann Weis

Physical Activity Readiness
Medical Examination for
Pregnancy

Advice for Active Living During Pregnancy

Pregnancy is a time when women can make beneficial changes in their health habits to protect and promote the healthy development of their unborn babies. These changes include adopting improved eating habits, abstinence from smoking and alcohol intake, and participating in regular moderate physical activity. Since all of these changes can be carried over into the postnatal period and beyond, pregnancy is a very good time to adopt healthy lifestyle habits that are permanent by integrating physical activity with enjoyable healthy eating and a positive self and body image.

Active Living:

- see your doctor before increasing your activity level during pregnancy
- exercise regularly but don't overexert
- exercise with a pregnant friend or join a prenatal exercise program
- follow FITT principles modified for pregnant women
- know safety considerations for exercise in pregnancy

Healthy Eating:

- the need for calories is higher (about 300 more per day) than before pregnancy
- follow Canada's Food Guide to Healthy Eating and choose healthy foods from the following groups: whole grain or enriched bread or cereal, fruits and vegetables, milk and milk products, meat, fish, poultry and alternatives
- drink 6-8 glasses of fluid, including water, each day
- salt intake should not be restricted
- limit caffeine intake i.e., coffee, tea, chocolate, and cola drinks
- dieting to lose weight is not recommended during pregnancy

Positive Self and Body Image:

- remember that it is normal to gain weight during pregnancy
- accept that your body shape will change during pregnancy
- enjoy your pregnancy as a unique and meaningful experience

For more detailed information and advice about pre- and postnatal exercise, you may wish to obtain a copy of a booklet entitled *Active Living During Pregnancy: Physical Activity Guidelines for Mother and Baby* © 1999. Available from the Canadian Society for Exercise Physiology, www.csep.ca. Cost: $11.95

Public Health Agency of Canada. The sensible guide to a healthy pregnancy. Minister of Health, 2012. Ottawa, Ontario K1A 0K9. http://www.phac-aspc.gc.ca/hp-gs/guide/assets/pdf/hpguide-eng.pdf. HC Pub.: 5830 Cat.: HP5-33/2012E. 1 800 O-Canada (1-800-622-6232) TTY: 1-800-926-9105.

Davenport MH. Charlesworth S. Vanderspank D. Sopper MM. Mottola MF. *Development and validation of exercise target heart rate zones for overweight and obese pregnant women.* Appl Physiol Nutr Metab. 2008; 33(5): 984-9.

Davies GAL. Wolfe LA. Mottola MF. MacKinnon C. *Joint SOGC / CSEP Clinical Practice Guidelines: Exercise in Pregnancy and the Postpartum Period.* Can J Appl Physiol. 2003; 28(3): 329-341.

Mottola MF, Davenport MH, Brun CR, Inglis SD, Charlesworth S, Sopper MM. *VO peak prediction and exercise prescription for pregnant women.* Med Sci Sports Exerc. 2006 Aug:38(8):1389-95.PMID: 16888450

SAFETY CONSIDERATIONS

- ◆ Avoid exercise in warm/humid environments, especially during the 1st trimester
- ◆ Avoid isometric exercise or straining while holding your breath
- ◆ Maintain adequate nutrition and hydration – drink liquids before and after exercise
- ◆ Avoid exercise while lying on your back past the 4th month of pregnancy
- ◆ Avoid activities which involve physical contact or danger of falling
- ◆ Know your limits – pregnancy is not a good time to train for athletic competition
- ◆ Know the reasons to stop exercise and consult a qualified health care provider immediately if they occur

REASONS TO STOP EXERCISE AND CONSULT YOUR HEALTH CARE PROVIDER

- ◆ Excessive shortness of breath
- ◆ Chest pain
- ◆ Painful uterine contractions (more than 6-8 per hour)
- ◆ Vaginal bleeding
- ◆ Any "gush" of fluid from vagina (suggesting premature rupture of the membranes)
- ◆ Dizziness or faintness

4

© Canadian Society for Exercise Physiology, 2013

APPENDIX 2

SAMPLE CARDIOVASCULAR WORKOUTS

Now that you are pregnant, does this mean that all your workouts need to be easy? Not necessarily. In fact, not only can you continue to sweat but you can also add some variety to your workouts. This is assuming of course, that you are having an uncomplicated pregnancy and that you have discussed your training and workouts with your doctor or midwife.

Below are 3 sample workouts that can be performed with most types of cardiovascular activities, including indoor cycling, running, swimming and elliptical. If you are not familiar with these types of workouts, we encourage waiting until your 2nd trimester before attempting them. In all cases, it is important to start off gradually and pay attention to how your body responds. Monitor your intensity by ensuring that:

- Your can carry on a conversation.
- Your heart rate does not go above the highest end of your prescribed heart rate training zone.
- Your rate of perceived exertion is within 12-14.

Workout #1: Modified Fartleks

- Start off with a gentle warm up (e.g. light spinning for 10 minutes).
- Spin slightly faster for 1 minute, while monitoring your intensity.
- Spin a bit easier for 1-2 minutes.
- Repeat steps 2 and 3 several times, while listening to your body and making sure that you are not exerting yourself too much.
- Finish off with a cool down (e.g. light spinning for 10 minutes).

Workout #2 Modified Tempo

- Start off with a gentle warm up (e.g. jogging or walking for 10 minutes).
- Pick up your pace slightly and hold it for 8-10 minutes, while monitoring your intensity.

- Slow your pace for 5 minutes.
- Repeat steps 2 and 3 (if desired).
- Finish off with a cool down (e.g. jogging or walking for 10 minutes).

Workout #3 Scramble Workout

- Start off with a gentle warm up (e.g. 10 minutes on the elliptical machine).
- Be creative and do something different every 2 minutes. For instance, stride forward, then stride backward, then stride forward while increasing the resistance and then stride easy for 2 minutes each. The point is simply to break up your workout, while still doing something that is a bit more challenging, while monitoring your intensity.
- Finish off with a cool down (e.g. less intensity on the elliptical for 10 minutes).

Although you may not reach the same level of intensity you were accustomed to prior to getting pregnant, you are still getting a great cardiovascular workout. These workouts will help maintain some of your pre-pregnancy fitness level and keep your workouts from getting stale. When planning such workouts, be sure to give your body adequate recovery time between the more intense sessions.

APPENDIX 3

YOGA POSES FOR THE PREGNANT ATHLETE

Below are a few simple poses that were selected with the pregnant athlete in mind. These poses can be done in your home, at the gym or even outside at the park. Consider meeting with a certified yoga instructor should you have further questions or if you are new to yoga.

Cat and Cow Pose: *Stretches back and shoulders and increases abdominal strength*

- Start on all fours, with your wrists underneath your shoulders and your knees underneath your hips. Ensure your spine remains neutral and engage your abdominal muscles while performing the movements.
- As you drop your belly toward the ground, slowly look up (cow). Start the movement with your tailbone, so that your neck is the last thing to move.
- Drop your head to look at your navel and round your spine up toward the ceiling (like a cat).
- Hold each pose for a few seconds.
- *Note:*
  - Think about moving each vertebrae one at a time as you lift your spine toward the ceiling or toward the ground.

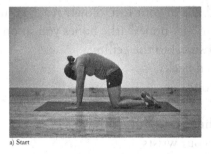
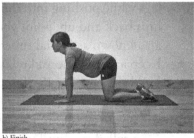

a) Start   b) Finish

Figure A3.0: Cat and Cow Pose

Child's Pose: *Stretches lower back, hips, thighs and ankles*

- Start on all fours, with your wrists underneath your shoulders, knees wider than your hips and heels wide apart and keep your big toes touching. This will allow space for your expanding belly.
- While keeping your hands where they are, try to sit on your heels, slowly sink your belly to your thighs and rest your forehead to the ground.
- Your arms should be in front of you with palms facing the floor. If you feel more comfortable, you can slide your arms back alongside your thighs with palms facing upwards. Relax your neck and shoulders.
- Hold the pose for 15-30 seconds.

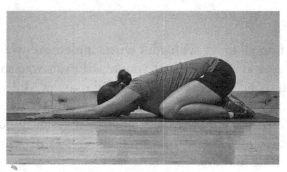

Figure A3.1: Child's Pose

Downward Dog: *Lengthens lower back, stretches shoulders and hamstrings*

- Start on all fours. Spread your fingers wide apart, extend them forward and keep them firm on the ground.
- As you exhale, lift your knees off the ground and straighten your legs while pushing into the balls of your feet. Slowly reach your hips back and up; point your "sits-bones" (the bones you sit on, also known as ischial tuberosities) to the ceiling.
- Keep a long spine and relaxed neck.
- Hold the pose for 15-30 seconds.
- *Note*:
  - If your wrists are sore while performing this yoga pose, place a rolled-up towel under your wrists.
  - If your hamstrings and/or lower back feel tight, bend your knees slightly.

Variation:

    ○ Place your hands on a chair (rather than on your mat) during your 3rd trimester.

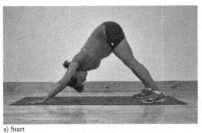
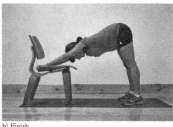

a) Start   b) Finish

Figure A3.2: Downward Dog

Squatting: *Opens pelvic area and strengthens legs for delivery*

- Stand with your feet slightly wider than your hips.
- Keep your heels on the floor, feet slightly turned out and bend your knees and hips as you lower yourself as close to the ground as possible. If necessary, use a sturdy table or chair in front of you to stabilize yourself while lowering.
- Hold this pose for 15-30 seconds.

Variation:

    ○ Place a small stool or several stacked phone books underneath your bottom to relieve some of the tension in your legs.
    ○ Clasp your hands together and push your elbows against the insides of your knees for an increased stretch.

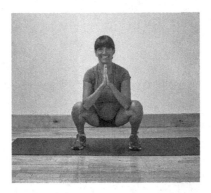

Figure A3.3: Squatting

225

APPENDIX 4

STRENGTHENING EXERCISES FOR THE PREGNANT ATHLETE

Listed below are a number of strengthening exercises that correspond with the suggestions found in the chapter "Cross Training Your Way Through Pregnancy". They are just a few of literally hundreds of exercises to help strengthen your body during pregnancy - and even into postpartum. We are not suggesting that you perform each of the following exercises in a single session. Rather, we provided many options to give you the freedom to pick and choose the exercises that work best for you. Just remember to incorporate several exercises according to the different areas of the body e.g. upper and lower body. These exercises can be done at the gym or at home, and some can be made more challenging by performing them on a BOSU or balance board. Ask a fitness professional for appropriate tips for this progression.

Keys to Strength Training Success:

- *Lift the correct weight.* Lift a weight that allows you to complete at least 10 but no more than 15 repetitions (reps) with maximum effort and proper form. Aim for 2 sets of each exercise.
- *Achieve muscle fatigue.* For optimal results, perform each set to the point of muscle fatigue (when your muscles are incapable of performing another rep in good form).
- *Progressive overload (Reps).* Begin with 10 reps and progress you way up to 15 reps on each and every set. Once you can perform 15 reps for both sets in good form, it is time to make the exercise more challenging by increasing the weight or resistance for that particular exercise.
- *Ensure proper technique.* With each and every exercise you want to complete the movement in a slow and controlled manner. Hold each exercise for a 1-2 count before returning to the start position.
- *Ask a fitness professional for help.* It is a good idea to seek help to ensure good form and lessen the risk of injury. In addition,

there are a wide variety of exercise machines at the gym that can be substituted for any of the exercises below. If you are unsure as to which machine to use or do not know how to work the machines in your facility, ask staff members for help.

- *Safety first.* Should you feel unstable while performing exercises on a ball or a BOSU, feel free to use a flat bench to complete these exercises. Alternatively, have someone spot you while doing such exercises.

LOWER BODY

Step-Ups

- Stand in front of a step. Place 1 foot firmly on the step and keep the other foot on the ground.
- Push through the heel that is on the step and straighten the knee and hip while lifting your other leg off the ground. Ensure to keep your knee over your 2nd toe.
- Slowly lower the leg and foot back to the ground and keep your foot on the step.

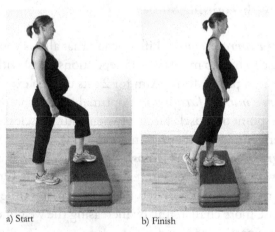

a) Start   b) Finish

Figure A4.0: Step-Ups

Squats

- Stand with your feet slightly wider than hip width apart, with your toes forward.
- Fold your arms across your chest. If balance is an issue, you can lift your arms and hands out in front to shoulder height.
- Bend at your knees and hips and lower your body until your thighs are parallel to the ground. Keep your chest pointed forward, to help maintain a neutral spine.
- Push through your heels, straighten your knees and hips into standing position and squeeze your glutes at the end of the movement.

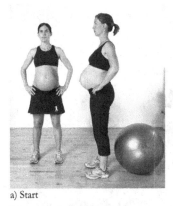 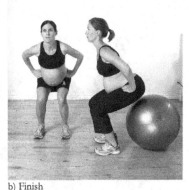

a) Start   b) Finish

Figure A4.1: Squats

Reverse Lunge and Forward Lunge

- Most lunge exercises are similar. Often they start and end in the same position with the difference occurring during the movement.
- Stand with your feet hip width apart and hands on your hips

Reverse Lunge	Front Lunge
• Take a large step back with 1 foot (approximately 1-2 feet). You should be on the ball of that foot.	• Take a large step forward with 1 foot (approximately 1-2 feet).

• Bend your back knee and lower it down until it almost touches the ground. • Your front knee should bend automatically and be aligned with your 2nd toe.	• Bend your back knee and lower it down until it almost touches the ground. • Your front knee should bend automatically and be aligned with your 2nd toe.
• Straighten your front leg as your back leg comes forward to meet the foot that is in front.	• Push through your front heel as you straighten your front knee and hip and step back to the foot that is behind.

- Repeat on the same leg for the appropriate number or reps and then switch to the other leg.

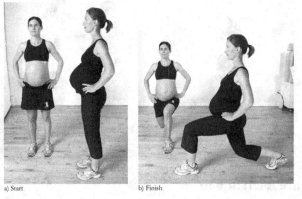

a) Start b) Finish

Figure A4.2: Reverse Lunge and Forward Lunge

Walking Lunges
- Stand with your feet hip width apart and hands on your hips.
- Take a large step forward with 1 foot. You should be on the ball of your foot of your back leg.
- Bend your back knee and lower it down until it almost touches the ground. Keep your front knee bent and aligned with your 2nd toe.
- "Walk" forward as you straighten your front knee and hip as you step your back leg past your front leg right into the next lunge.

- Repeat for 10-15 steps on each leg to complete 1 set.
- Refer to Reverse Lunge and Forward Lunge pictures.

Squat Plus Woodchop

- Stand with your feet slightly wider than hip width apart, toes forward.
- Hold a medicine ball close to your abdomen.
- Bend at your knees and hips and lower your body until your thighs are parallel to the ground.
- Lower the ball to the outside of 1 thigh. As you stand up, lift the ball across the body and over the opposite shoulder.
- As you return to the squat position, lower the ball back to the outside of the opposite thigh again.
- *Note:*
  - You should not perform this exercise if you have Diastasis Recti.

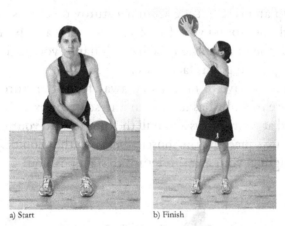

a) Start   b) Finish

Figure A4.3: Squat Plus Woodchop

Lying Hamstring Curl Off Ball

- Lie on your back with your legs straight and heels on an exercise ball. Hands can be at your side for support.
- Balance your heels on the ball while you lift your hips off the ground.

- Bend your knees to roll the ball toward you until your feet are flat on the ball.
- Keep your hips high, straighten your legs and roll the ball back to almost start position.

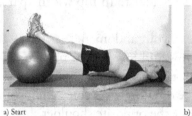 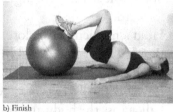

a) Start   b) Finish

Figure A4.4: Lying Hamstring Curl Off Ball

UPPER BODY

Row with Exercise Tube

- Wrap an exercise tube around a sturdy object just above waist height or around your feet if you are in a seated position.
- Grab the ends of the tube in each hand; your arms should be straight and palms facing each other.
- You may have to take a step away from the sturdy object to ensure the tube has tension in it to start the exercise.
- Bend at your elbows and pull the tube toward your waist; ensure you are squeezing the muscles between the shoulder blades.
- Straighten your arms to return to start position.

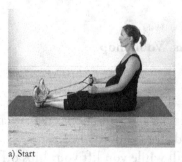 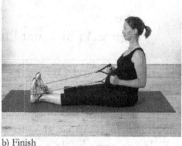

a) Start   b) Finish

Figure A4.5: Row with Exercise Tube

Rhomboid Squeeze

- Grab the ends of the band in each hand. Arms should be at shoulder height and palms face down.
- Ensure that the band has tension and your arms are straight.
- Bend at your elbows and pull the exercise band toward your shoulders and ensure that you squeeze your shoulder blades together.
- Straighten your arms again.

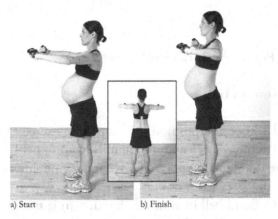

a) Start   b) Finish

Figure A4.6: Rhomboid Squeeze

Lat Pull Down

- Stand tall with your feet about hip width apart. Hold the ends of the exercise band in both hands above your head. Hands are a bit wider than shoulder width apart.
- Ensure the band has tension and your arms are straight.
- Bend your elbows and bring the band down to the top of your chest.
- Straighten the arms back over your head.

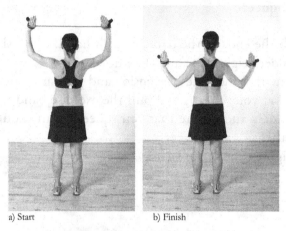

a) Start   b) Finish

Figure A4.7: Lat Pull Down

Bent Over Row on Ball

- Bend 1 knee and position it on top of an exercise ball.
- Bend at the waist, lean forward until your upper body is parallel to the floor and supported by 1 hand (same side as the knee on the ball).
- Hold a dumbbell in your free hand, arm is straight down with palm facing the ball.
- Bend at the elbow, pull the weight toward your shoulder and keep your body as still as possible.
- Slowly lower the arm back down again.

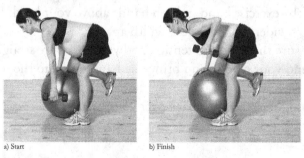

a) Start   b) Finish

Figure A4.8: Bent Over Row on Ball

Modified Push-Up

- Kneel on the floor and walk your hands forward until your body is in a straight line at a 45° angle to the ground.
- Your arms should be straight with your hands slightly wider than shoulder width apart.
- Bend your elbows outward and lower your entire body down until your nose almost touches the ground.
- Straighten your arms and return to start position.

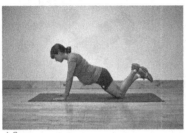 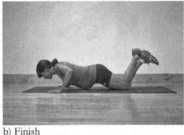

a) Start   b) Finish

Figure A4.9: Modified Push-Up

Regular Push-Up

- This push-up is similar to the push-up with bent knees however your starting position is on your hands and toes.

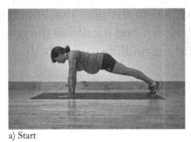 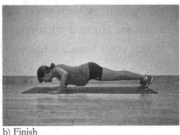

a) Start   b) Finish

Figure A4.10: Push-Up

Incline Press Off the Ball

- Sit on an exercise ball, slowly roll yourself down until the ball is at the level of your shoulders and your body is at a 45° angle.

- With a dumbbell in each hand, bring your hands close to your shoulders and your palms face forward.
- Push your arms up and toward the mid-line of your body until the weights almost touch.
- Lower your arms down slowly until your hands return to your shoulders.

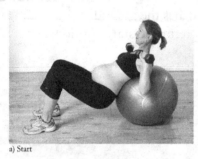 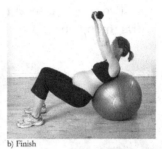

a) Start   b) Finish

Figure A4.11: Incline Press

Chest Flyes Off the Ball

- Sit on an exercise ball and slowly roll down until your head and upper back are supported on the ball.
- With a dumbbell in each hand, straighten your arms above your chest, palms facing each other.
- Your elbows should be slightly bent while performing the movement. Open your arms (out to the side) until the upper arms are aligned with your shoulders and parallel to the ground.
- Bring your hands back toward the midline of your body.

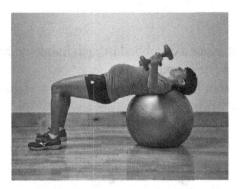

Figure A4.12: Chest Flyes Off the Ball

Lateral Raise

- Stand tall, place a dumbbell in each hand, arms are straight down by the side of your body and palms face the side of your thighs.
- Lift your arms out to the side until they are at shoulder height.
- Your elbows should remain slightly bent while performing this movement.
- Slowly lower your arms back down to start position.

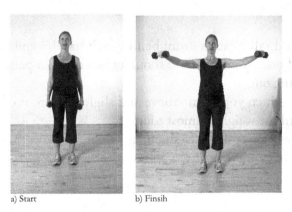

a) Start   b) Finsih

Figure A4.13: Lateral Raise

Front Raise

- Stand tall, place a dumbbell in each hand and arms are straight down, in front of your thighs.
- Lift 1 arm out in front to shoulder height and slowly lower down.
- Alternate arms.

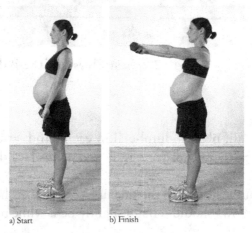

a) Start   b) Finish

Figure A4.14: Front Raise

Shoulder Press

- Stand tall, place a dumbbell in each hand, bend your elbows and bring your hands to shoulder height. Your palms should be facing out.
- Straighten your arms above and slightly in front of your head, until the weights almost touch.
- Slowly lower down to shoulder height.

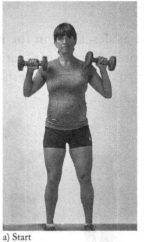 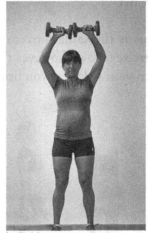

a) Start   b) Finish

Figure A4.15: Shoulder Press

Bicep Curl with Exercise Tube

- Stand tall, place the tube under the feet and a handle in each hand, arms are straight down by the side of your body and palms face the side of your thighs.
- Keep your upper arms at your side and bend the elbows while turning your palms toward your shoulders.
- Straighten your arms back down toward your thighs.

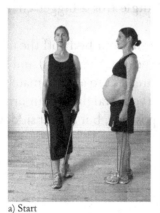 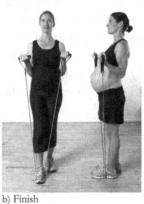

a) Start   b) Finish

Figure A4.16: Bicep Curl

Hammer Curl

- This is the same movement as described in the Bicep Curl exercise (above) however the only difference is that you do not turn your palms as you bring your hands to your shoulders.

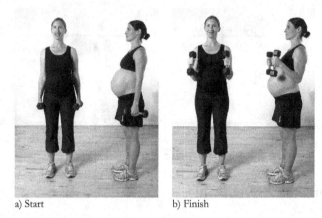

a) Start   b) Finish

Figure A4.17: Hammer Curl

Dips Off a Chair (or Bench)

- Sit on the edge of a chair (or bench) with your hands at your side and palms flat on the bench, fingers point toward your knees.
- Bend your knees to a 90° angle (for a bigger challenge, try straightening your legs).
- Straighten your arms as your lift your body off the table.
- Keep your backside close to the chair (or bench) and lower your body down until your arms are bent to approximately 90°.
- Push through your hands as you straighten your arms and lift your torso back to the start position, but do not sit down.

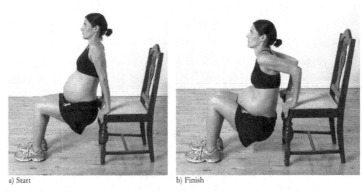

a) Start   b) Finish

Figure A4.18: Dips Off a Chair (or Bench)

Overhead Tricep Extension Seated on a Ball

- Sit on an exercise ball with a dumbbell in 1 hand and your arm extended over your head. Keep your upper arm close to your ear.
- Without moving your upper arms, bend at your elbow and lower the dumbbell toward your shoulder blades.
- Slowly straighten your arm back to the start position.

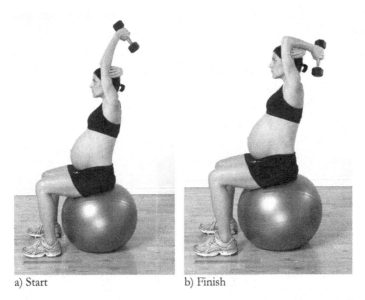

a) Start   b) Finish

Figure A4.19: Overhead Tricep Extension Seated on a Ball

APPENDIX 5

My Food Guide Servings Tracker   NAME: _____   DATE: _____

Food Guide Servings per day

PREGNANT FEMALE AGED 19–50

○ 7–8   **Vegetables and Fruit**

1 Food Guide Serving =
125 mL (½ cup) fresh, frozen or canned vegetable or fruit or 100% juice or
250 mL (1 cup) leafy raw vegetables or salad or
1 piece of fruit

○ 6–7   **Grain Products**

1 Food Guide Serving =
1 slice (35 g) of bread or ½ pita or tortilla (35 g) or
125 mL (½ cup) cooked rice, pasta or couscous or
30 g cold cereal or 175 mL (¾ cup) hot cereal

○ 2   **Milk and Alternatives**

1 Food Guide Serving =
250 ml (1 cup) milk or fortified soy beverage or
175 g (¾ cup) yogurt or
50 g (1 ½ oz) cheese

○ 2   **Meat and Alternatives**

1 Food Guide Serving =
75 g (2 ½ oz)/125 mL (½ cup) cooked fish, shellfish, poultry or lean meat or
175 mL (¾ cup) cooked legumes or tofu or
60 mL (¼ cup) shelled nuts and seeds

2–3   Include an extra 2 to 3 Food Guide Servings from any of the four food groups each day.

30 to 45 mL (2 to 3 Tbsp) each day   **Oils and Fats**
Include a small amount of unsaturated fat each day. This includes oil used for cooking, salad dressings, margarine and mayonnaise.

☐ Include a multivitamin containing folic acid and iron every day.
☐ Eat at least one dark green and one orange vegetable each day.
☐ Choose vegetables and fruit prepared with little or no added fat, sugar or salt.
☐ Have vegetables and fruit more often than juice.
☐ Make at least half of your grain products whole grain each day.
☐ Choose grain products that are lower in fat, sugar or salt.
☐ Drink skim, 1% or 2% milk each day.
☐ Select lower fat milk alternatives.
☐ Have meat alternatives such as beans, lentils and tofu often.
☐ Eat at least two Food Guide Servings of fish each week.
☐ Select lean meat and alternatives prepared with little or no added fat or salt.
☐ Satisfy your thirst with water.
☐ Limit foods and beverages high in calories, fat, sugar or salt.
☐ Be active every day as part of a healthy pregnancy. See your doctor before increasing your activity level.

For more information and to order copies of Canada's Food Guide visit Canada's Food Guide on line.

www.healthcanada.gc.ca/foodguide

Canada

APPENDIX 6

BIRTH PREPARATION ROUTINE
The following exercises will help you activate and coordinate your abdominal and pelvic floor muscles to facilitate childbirth. Learning to work these muscles in tandem will mimic what you are trying to achieve during labour. We suggest working on the abdominal and the pelvic floor muscle exercises *separately*, prior to bringing the 2 parts together. It is recommended that you first read the chapter "Your Silent Training Partner - Your Pelvic Floor Muscles" to review how to perform the pelvic floor strengthening exercises correctly.

You will be working through 4 different stages, so it is best to start as early as possible. No worries if you are receiving this information late in your pregnancy, as it is never too late to start. There is no correct amount of time that you should spend at each stage; the progression is based on your own comfort level. We suggest breaking up the stages into 4 equal time lines that correspond to the remaining number of weeks until your due date. For instance, if you are currently in your 20th week, you can work on each stage for approximately 5 weeks.

Below is the description of the Birth Preparation Routine. All exercises can be performed seated, lying down or standing. Aim for 2-3 sets per day.

Stage 1:

Abdominal Exercise
- Practice pulling your belly button in (like when you are anticipating a blow to the stomach). Hold for a 1-2 count.
- Release and repeat 10-15 times.

Pelvic Floor Exercise
- Perform the basic contraction exercise as described in the chapter "Your Silent Training Partner – Your Pelvic Floor Muscles". Pull the pelvic floor muscles up and hold for a 1-2 count.
- Release and repeat 10-15 times.

Stage 2:

Abdominal Exercise
- Take a deep breath in and let your belly go (e.g. do not hold or suck your belly in).
- As you breathe out, pull your belly button in as though you are giving your baby a hug from the inside.
- Hold your hug for 10 seconds. You will need to modify your breathing so that you can breathe without letting the hug go.
- Release and repeat many times throughout the day.

Stage 3:

Abdominal Exercise
- Take a deep breath in and let your belly go.
- As you breathe out, pull your belly button in as though you are giving your baby a hug from the inside.
- Hold your hug for 20-30 seconds. You will need to modify your breathing so that you can breathe without letting the hug go. Rest assured, you are not harming your baby.
- Release and repeat this exercise many times throughout the day.

Pelvic Floor Exercise
- You are still riding the elevator, but now you want to teach your pelvic floor muscles to relax completely and "go into the basement".
- The goal is to ensure you have enough control over your pelvic floor muscles and can relax them almost on command. You will need this technique when it comes time to push.
- Attempt this exercise many times throughout the day.

You and your partner may want to use the words "go into the basement" (or something more to your liking) as a key phrase during labour. This will help to recognize when you need to relax the pelvic floor muscles and push.

Stage 4:

Bringing the 2 Exercises Together
- You are now going to practice putting these 2 exercises together and mimic what you will be doing in labour: contracting (or engaging) the abdominals while also releasing the pelvic floor muscles "into the basement".
- Take a deep breath in and let your belly go.
- As you breathe out, pull your belly button in and squeeze your pelvic floor muscles up.
- While you are holding your belly button in, release your pelvic floor muscles "into the basement".
- Aim to do this for 10-15 seconds.
- Attempt to do this exercise many times throughout the day.

Remember that this coordination between your abdominal and pelvic floor muscles will not necessarily happen automatically. Similar to any other muscle needed to perform an intense activity, you will have to train these muscles before they can benefit you in the delivery room.

Pelvic Floor Exercise
- Perform the elevator exercise described in the chapter "Your Silent Training Partner – Your Pelvic Floor Muscles". You can either go straight up and down the floors or you can add in some variation by mixing up the floors. You do not have to worry about "going into the basement" yet.
- Attempt this exercise many times throughout the day.

APPENDIX 7

STOP BREAKING YOUR (UPPER) BACK, BABY!

You will be bending over your little one countless times during the day –while changing diapers, putting him or her into their crib, feeding and just loving them. These actions could contribute toward postural imbalances, specifically your upper back and neck. An easy rule of thumb to correct postural imbalances is to lengthen the muscles that are tight and strengthen the muscles that are weak. These 3 simple exercises can be done every day at home to help combat your aches and pains.

Keys To Upper Back and Neck Strengthening Success:

- *Progressive overload (Sets & Reps).* Begin with 10 repetitions (reps) and progress you way up to 15 reps on each and every set. You want to aim for 2-3 sets of each exercise. Once you can perform 15 reps for both sets in good form, it is time to make the exercise more challenging by increasing the weight or resistance for that particular exercise.
- *Progressive overload (Timed).* There are some exercises listed below which are timed. Start out by holding the exercise for 10 seconds. Over each session, work your way to 60-90 seconds. Aim to complete 2-3 sets of these exercises.
- *Achieve muscle fatigue.* For optimal results, perform each set to the point of muscle fatigue (when your muscles are incapable of performing another rep in good form).
- *Ensure proper technique.* With each and every exercise you want to complete the movement in a slow and controlled manner. For most exercises listed below, you want to hold each exercise for a 1-2 count before returning to the start position.
- *Ask a fitness professional for help.* It is a good idea to seek help to ensure good form and lessen the risk of injury. In addition, there are a variety of exercises that can further strengthen your

mid-back; ask a fitness professional for help if you are unsure about the exercises.

Stretching Your Chest Muscles
- Stand in a doorway.
- Bend 1 arm and shoulder to about 90° and place it on the frame of a doorway.
- Once your arm is secure, turn your body away from your arm until you feel a stretch in the chest area.
- Switch arms.
- Hold this stretch 30-60 seconds on each side.

Strengthen Your Midback Muscles
- Scapular retraction – also known as "setting the scapula".
- You are trying to strengthen the muscles around the shoulder blades (also known as scapula), so you want to try and think about those muscles while performing these exercises.
- Draw the lower part of the shoulder blades down your back, as though you are trying to put them into the back pocket of your jeans.
- Then, without using your upper back or shoulder muscles, squeeze the shoulder blades gently together. Think about squeezing a pencil between your shoulder blades.
- This is a very subtle movement; do not get frustrated if you do not get the movement right away.

Strengthen Your Deep Neck Muscles and Lengthen Your Small Neck Muscles
- Lie on your back so that you are comfortable and your legs are extended.
- Your neck should be in neutral position (e.g. maintaining the curve in your neck).
- Without lifting your head, tuck your chin into your chest and hold for a 3-5 second count. You will likely feel a stretch in the back of the neck and/or down your back.
- Return your head back to neutral position.

As stated above, you can always consult a fitness or health care provider to check your form and technique. In addition, they may suggest other therapies, such as massage, acupuncture or spinal manipulation to help relieve your aches and pains.

APPENDIX 8

CORE STRENGTHENING EXERCISES

Listed below are a number of strengthening exercises that correspond to the suggestions found in the chapter "Your Strong And Powerful Core". We have incorporated enough variety to ensure that you are challenging your core without boredom setting in. Have fun!

Keys to Core Strengthening Success:

- *Belly breathe baby!* Take note of the first exercise described below, as it is important to belly breathe with all exercises to ensure that your abdominals are engaged and supporting your core.
- *Lift the correct weight.* Lift a weight that allows you to complete at least 10 but no more than 15 repetitions (reps) with maximum effort and proper form. Aim for 2 sets of each exercise.
- *Achieve muscle fatigue.* For optimal results, perform each set to the point of muscle fatigue (when your muscles are incapable of performing another rep in good form).
- *Progressive overload (Reps).* For most exercises listed below, you may progress from 10 up to 15 reps, aiming for 15 reps on each and every set. Once you can perform 15 reps in good form, it is time to increase the weight for that particular exercise.
- *Progressive overload (Timed).* There are some exercises listed below which are timed. Start out by performing a modified version of the exercise (to ensure good form) and hold the exercise for 10 seconds. Over each session, work your way to 60 seconds. Once you can complete 2 sets of 60 seconds, move on to a more challenging version of the exercise.
- *Ask a fitness professional for help.* It is a good idea to seek help to ensure good form and lessen the risk of injury.
- *Safety first.* Should you feel unstable while performing exercises on a ball or a BOSU, feel free to use a flat bench to complete these exercises. Alternatively, have someone spot you while doing such exercises.

INITIAL EXERCISES

Baby Hugs (Belly Breathing)

- Stand or sit tall; maintain a neutral spine by keeping the curves in your neck and lower back.
- As you inhale, take a deep breath in and "let your belly go". You should see your stomach rise.
- As you exhale, draw your belly button in as far as you can. Maintain the curves in your back and neck. In other words, don't collapse your back.
- Hold your abdominals in for a 3-4 count and as you inhale, release slowly.
- Repeat 10-15 times.
- *Note:*
  - This exercise can be performed lying down as well. Always maintain a neutral spine. If you are attempting this exercise lying down while pregnant and feel dizzy, discontinue the exercise and try another exercise in the list.
  - It is a good idea to belly breathe with all exercises to ensure that your abdominals are engaged and supporting your core.

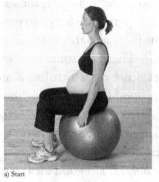 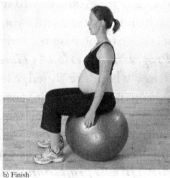

a) Start b) Finish

Figure A8.0: Baby Hugs

Ball Curls

- Sit on an exercise ball and roll down on the ball until it is positioned under your low back.
- Place your hands on your head or across your chest. Your jaw and neck should be relaxed.
- As you breathe in, let your belly go (or expand). As you start to breathe out, pull your belly button to your spine and lift your head and shoulders away from the ball.
- As you breathe in, let your belly go and lower your head and shoulders toward the ball.
- Repeat 10-15 times.

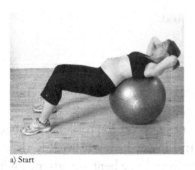 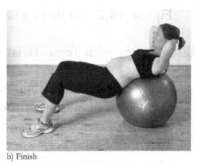

a) Start   b) Finish

Figure A8.1: Ball Curls

Single Leg ¼ Squat

- Stand tall and face a mirror and place your hands on your hips. Stand on 1 leg and ensure that your hips are at the same height.
- Bend the knee and hip of your standing leg, as though you are curtseying to the Queen. Ensure that your knee does not drop in or to the outside of your 2nd toe.
- Extend your hip and knee back to standing position.
- Repeat 10-15 times and then do the other leg.
- *Variation:*
  - You can hold onto a chair if you have trouble balancing.
  - Standing on a pillow can make this exercise more challenging.

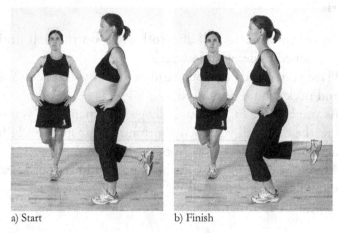

a) Start   b) Finish

Figure A8.2: Single Leg ¼ Squat

Walking Lunge with Torso Twist

- Stand tall, keep your abdominals engaged, and hold a weight or medicine ball in front of you, arms bent at 90°.
- Take a big step forward and come up on the toes of your back foot. Bend your back knee and lower it down until it almost touches the ground. Keep your front knee bent and aligned with your 2nd toe.
- While in this position, pause for a moment and turn your arms and torso in one direction (e.g. to the right) and then to the other (e.g. to the left).
- "Walk" forward as you straighten your front knee and hip as you step your back leg past your front leg right into the next lunge.
- Repeat 10-15 lunges on each leg.
- *Note:*
  - Avoid using a weight if you feel off balance while doing this exercise.

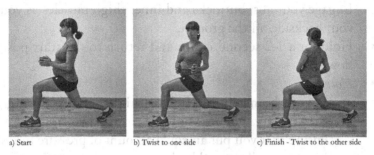

a) Start   b) Twist to one side   c) Finish - Twist to the other side

Figure A8.3: Walking Lunge with Torso Twist

Hip Hikes

- Stand sideways with 1 leg on a stair or bench; your other foot should hover just off the step, close to the edge. Keep both hips level.
- Keep your standing leg straight and lower the opposite leg down as though you are trying to touch the stair or ground below you. Your hips should no longer be even.
- Return the hips to an even position.
- Repeat 10-20 times on each leg.

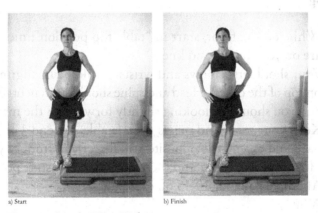

a) Start   b) Finish

Figure A8.4: Hip Hikes

Bridge

- Lie on your back with your knees and hips bent, feet on the ground; ankles, knees and hips are in alignment.

- Engage your abs, buttocks and inner thigh muscles as you lift your backside off the ground.
- Hold for a 1-2 second count and return to the start position slowly.
- *Note:*
  - If your hamstrings (back of thighs) cramp during this exercise, try moving your feet closer to your body and/or ensure that you put an equal amount of pressure into your big toe, small toe and heel.

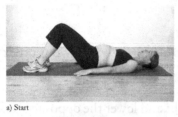 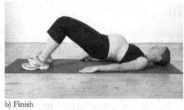

a) Start   b) Finish

Figure A8.5: Bridge

PROGRESSION EXERCISES

Bird Dog

- While on the floor, start in "table top position"; meaning you are on your hands and knees.
- Your shoulders, elbows and wrists should be in alignment (one on top of the other). Head and spine should be in neutral position and you should be looking slightly forward on the mat.
- Keep your torso and pelvis even (stable), extend 1 leg directly back and extend the opposite arm directly in front of you.
- Hold for a 1-2 count and then lower down to start position.
- Alternate pairs for 10-15 on each side.
- *Note:*
  - If this exercise places too much pressure on your wrist, try rolling a towel under your wrists. Otherwise, discontinue this exercise and continue with the bridge exercise described above.

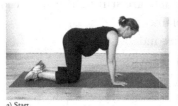 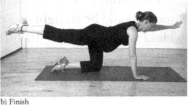

a) Start   b) Finish

Figure A8.6: Bird Dog

- *Variations:*
  - Single leg:
    - Same start position as above. Extend 1 leg back, hold for a 1-2 count and lower down slowly. Alternate legs, 10-15 each side.
  - Single arm:
    - Same start position as above. Extend 1 arm in front of you, hold for a 1-2 count and lower down slowly. Alternate arms, 10-15 each side.
  - Modified bird dog:
    - Same starting position as above. Extend your arm and leg along the ground and bring them back to start position. Alternate pairs, 10-15 each side.
  - Once you have progressed through the 3 variations above, try performing the original bird dog detailed above.

Side Plank

- Lie on your side and keep your elbow in line with your shoulder. The other arm can be on your waist or bent in front of the chest with your hand resting on the opposite shoulder.
- The sides of your feet can either be stacked on top of each other or kept slightly apart on the ground.
- Breathe in and let your belly go. As you breathe out and pull your belly in, lift your torso off the ground. Support yourself on your elbow and your feet.

- Ensure your elbow and shoulders are still in alignment. Your torso should be straight as a plank.
- Hold this position for 10-60 seconds.

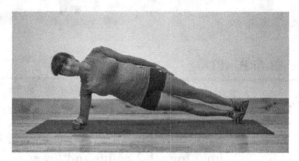

Figure A8.7: Side Plank

- *Variations:* If your back starts to hurt with this position, try the variations listed below. Aim to hold these positions for 10-60 seconds and complete 2 sets. Repeat on each side. Progress to a harder position once you can perform both sets for 60 seconds.
  - Leaning against the wall:
    - Bend the elbow closest to the wall up to shoulder height and lean it against the wall. Take a step away from the wall so that your body is at 45° from it.
  - Lowering yourself to a counter:
    - As you get stronger, you can lower yourself down closer to the ground. Find a counter or bed and bend your elbow to 90°, feet straight out from the counter. You are supporting your body on your elbow and side of feet.
  - On the ground with bent knees:
    - Same position as a side plank on the ground *except* instead of your legs being stretched out, bend at your knees. This way you are lifting up your body with the anchor points being the shoulder and knees.
  - Once you have progressed through the 3 variations above, try performing the original side plank described above.

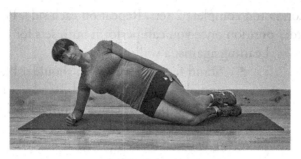

Figure A8.8: Modified Side Plank

Plank

- Lie face down, with both of your elbows bent at 90° and hands out in front.
- Curl your toes under, so that your toes and ankles are in alignment.
- Breathe in and let your belly go. As you breathe out and pull your abs in, lift your torso off the ground onto your toes and elbows. Make sure to keep your abdominal muscles engaged so that you are using your core and not your shoulders to maintain proper form and keep torso straight.
- If your back starts to hurt, lift the hips a little higher. If this does not alleviate the pain, lower down, take a break and try in a few minutes.
- Hold this position for 10-60 seconds.

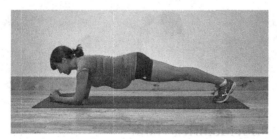

Figure A8.9: Plank

- *Variations:* If your back starts to hurt with this position, try the variations listed below. Aim to hold these positions for 10-60 seconds and complete 2 sets. Repeat on each side. Progress to a harder position once you can perform both sets for 60 seconds.

- o Leaning against a wall:
  - ▪ Stand facing a wall with shoulder blades down and abdominals engaged. Bend your elbows at 90° and place them at shoulder height on the wall.
- o Lowering yourself to a counter:
  - ▪ As you get stronger, you can lower yourself down closer to the ground. Find a counter or bed and bend your elbows to 90°, feet straight out from the counter (you will likely be on your tiptoes).
- o On the ground with bent knees:
  - ▪ Same position as described above in plank on the ground *except* lower onto your knees rather than extending your legs back. This way you are lifting up your body with the anchor points being the shoulders and knees.
- o Once you have progressed through the 3 variations above, try performing the original plank described above.

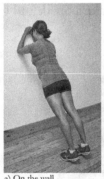 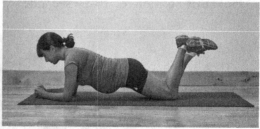

a) On the wall   b) On the ground

Figure A8.10: Modified Plank

Squats Off a BOSU

- • Place a BOSU on the ground with the flat side down.

- Step onto the BOSU with your feet equal distance apart and toes point forward. Ensure that you have your balance prior to starting the exercise.
- Fold your arms across your chest. However, if balance is an issue, you can lift your arms and hands out in front to shoulder height.
- Bend at your knees and hips and lower your body until your thighs are parallel to the ground. Keep your chest pointed forward, to help maintain a neutral spine.
- Push through your heels, straighten your knees and hips into standing position and squeeze your glutes at the end of the movement.
- Repeat 10-15 times.

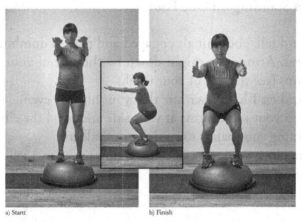

a) Startt   b) Finish

Figure A8.11: Squat

Lunging on Top of a BOSU

- Place the BOSU about 3-4 feet in front of you, with the flat side down.
- Stand tall, abdominals engaged and your shoulders down.
- Take a step forward so that 1 foot lands on the top of the BOSU and you come up on your back toes.
- Bend your back knee and lower it down until it almost touches the ground. Keep your front knee bent and aligned with your 2nd toe.
- Straighten your front knee and hip as you step your front leg off the BOSU and next to the standing leg.
- Repeat 10-15 times.

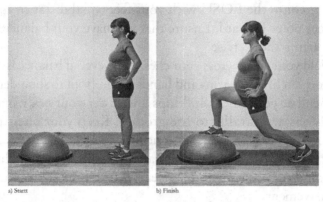

a) Startt   b) Finish

Figure A8.12: Lunging on Top of a BOSU

Bicep Curl Standing on One Foot

- Stand tall, abdominals engaged and place a dumbbell in each hand. Arms are straight down by the side of your body and palms face the side of your thighs.
- Stand on 1 leg and ensure that your hips are even.
- Keep your upper arms at your side and bend the elbows while turning your palms toward your shoulders.
- Straighten your arms back down toward your thighs.
- Repeat 10-15 times.

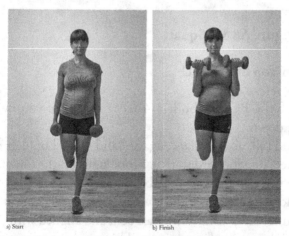

a) Start   b) Finish

Figure A8.13: Bicep Curl While Standing on One Foot

Shoulder Press Standing on a BOSU

- Place a BOSU on the ground with the flat side down.
- Step onto the BOSU with your feet equal distance apart. Ensure that you have your balance prior to starting the exercise.
- Place a dumbbell in each hand, bend at your elbows so that your palms are facing out and are at shoulder height.
- Extend the arms above your head but slightly in front, until the weights almost touch.
- Return your hands to your shoulders.
- Repeat 10-15 times.

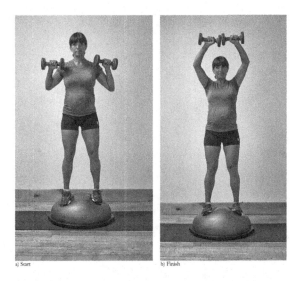

a) Start   b) Finish

Figure A8.14: Shoulder Press While Standing on a BOSU

OUR ALL-STAR TEAM

OUR ALL-STAR TEAM

This book would not have been possible without the information, advice and personal stories from our amazing team. To the talented and passionate athletes, thank you for sharing your stories and inspiring other women. To the clinicians, researchers and health and fitness professionals, thank you for sharing your expertise and knowledge and for guiding us in our writing.

Our Athletes

Alisa Bridgman is a runner, recent triathlete, former competitive alpine skier and mother of 3. She ran the Boston Marathon, placed 4th in her age category at the 2014 Subaru Niagara Triathlon and has a personal best of 3:38:38 for the marathon.

Allison Chisholm is a triathlete and mother of 2. She received several gold and silver medals at the Police Fire World Games in 2008 and 2010 while competing in the time trial, hill climb, road bike and triathlon events. She placed 2nd at the 2013 Toronto Triathlon Festival and 33rd in her age category at the 2013 World Championship Triathlon Olympic distance.

Amy Lyman Nedeau is a long distance runner and mother of 1. She was a 2000 Olympic Trials Track Finalist in the 1500m event and awarded the NCAA Division I All American Track and Field.

Annette Carling is triathlete and mother of 1. She completed the 2010 Ironman Lake Placid and the 2012 Ironman 70.3 Mont Tremblant. She is also one of the models in our book, including the image on the front cover.

Belinda Bain is a cyclist and mother of 2. She placed 2nd in her age category at the 2013 Collingwood Centurion and won her age category at the 2011 Guelph Lake Triathlon.

Christiane Tremblay is a triathlete, runner and mother of 4. She completed the 2013 Ironman 70.3 Mont-Tremblant and the 2014

Ironman 70.3 New Orleans. She completed numerous running events from 5K to 21.1K.

Christine Wallace is triathlete, runner and mother of 2. She raced the 2012 Ironman 70.3 Miami (4:59:54). She has personal bests of 18:59 for 5K and 10:29 for 3000m event.

Danelle Kabush is a professional XTERRA triathlete and mother of 2. She is a member of the Luna Pro Team and won a bronze medal in 2004 and silver medals at the 2006 and 2008 XTERRA World Championships. Follow her blog "Adventures in Balancing Motherhood with Racing" at www.danellekabush.com.

Deborah Moore is a triathlete and mother of 3. She raced the 2007 Ford Ironman 70.3 World Championship and the 2005 Ford Ironman World Championship. She placed top 10 in her age category at the 2003 and 2005 Ironman Lake Placid.

Fiona Whitby is a triathlete, runner and mother of 1. She races professionally and has numerous top 10 finishes, including Ironman events.

Fulvia Manarin is a runner and mother of 3. She ran the 2014 Boston Marathon (3:32:08) and the 2013 Hamilton Marathon (3:32:38).

Heather Lowe is a triathlete and mother of 2. She completed the 2009 Ironman Canada and the 2011 Ironman Lake Placid.

Jaclyn Kissel is a former sprinter, triathlete, runner and mother of 1. She was captain of the McMaster track and field team and competed as a sprinter at the Canadian Inter University Sport National Meet. She placed 2nd overall and 1st in her age category at the 2010 Ontario's Women's Only Triathlon and 3rd in her age category at the 2012 Subaru Orillia Triathlon.

Jean Wilson is a runner and mother of 1. She won the 2013 Dublin Master's Cross Country Championship, received a silver medal at the 2007 Dublin Senior Cross Country Championship and won the 2006 National Novice Cross Country Championship.

Jennifer Drynan is a distance runner and mother of 2. She placed 2nd at both the 2013 Niagara Falls International Marathon (2:49:51) and the 2003 Scotiabank Toronto Waterfront half marathon (1:18:32).

Jennifer Young is a triathlete, runner and mother of 2. She placed 1st at the 2014 MEC 15K run (1:11: 33) and completed the 2003 Ironman Canada (11:47:25).

Jessica Adam is a triathlete and mother of 2. She won the Canadian Triathlon Championship in her age category, placed 6th in her age category at the 2008 World Triathlon Championship and completed the 2009 Ironman Canada.

Jessica Zelinka is a Canadian Olympic heptathlete, 100m hurdler and mother of 1. She won silver at the 2014 Commonwealth Games, competed in the 2012 & 2008 summer Olympics and won gold at the 2007 Pan American Games.

Karen Cockburn is a Canadian Olympic trampolinist. She is a 3-time Olympic medalist, winning silver medals in 2004 and 2008 and a bronze medal in 2000. She placed 4th at the 2012 Olympic Games. She was the World Champion at the 2007 Pan Am Games.

Karen Soos is a marathoner and mother of 3. She raced numerous events, placed 5th in her age category at the 2014 Toronto Women's Half Marathon and will be running the 2015 Boston Marathon.

Kathie Howes is a runner, triathlete and mother of 2. She raced the 2008 and 2009 Ironman Lake Placid and placed 4th in her age category at the 2012 Guelph Lake II Duathlon.

Kelley Cullen is an off-road triathlete and mother of 2. She won the bronze medal at the 2013 XTERRA Mountain Championship, gold medal at the 2011 XTERRA Indian Peaks and placed 4th at the 2011 XTERRA USA Championship.

Krista DuChene is a professional runner and mother of 3. She is the second fastest Canadian female marathoner (2:28:32), won the 2013

Scotiabank Vancouver Half Marathon (1:10:52) and represented Canada at the 2013 World Marathon Championship.

Leslie Black is a runner, triathlete and mother of 4. She placed 2nd in her age category at the 2014 Ironman 70.3 World Championship, won the 2013 Toronto Half Marathon and placed 3rd at the 2012 Sporting Life 10K.

Lucia Mahoney is a runner and mother of 3. She ran the Boston Marathon 3 times and frequently wins her age category in races. Her personal best marathon time is 3:12:44.

Mary Davies is a professional runner and mother of 2. She won the 2012 Scotiabank Toronto Waterfront Marathon (2:28:56) and represented New Zealand at the 2009 and 2013 World Championships.

Morgan is a competitive swimmer and mother of 2. She was awarded the United States Swimming Scholastic All-American and was a member of the Harvard Varsity Swim Team.

Priscilla Lopes-Schliep is a Canadian Olympic Hurdler and mother of 2. She won a bronze medal (100MH) at the 2008 Summer Olympics, a silver medal (100MH) at the 2009 World Championship and a bronze medal (60MH) at the 2010 Indoor World Championship. She won the inaugural Diamond League Championship in 2010 and was the fastest hurdler in the world the same year.

Seana Zelazo is marathon runner and mother of 1. She is a 2-time marathon Olympic trials qualifier (2004 and 2008), won the 2003 Philadelphia Marathon (2:45:05) and finished 4th at the 2007 Hartford Marathon.

Seanna Keating is a squash player and mother of 3. She was the 2011 Double Squash World Champion and placed top 10 in Canadian singles for over 10 years.

Seanna Robinson is a runner and mother of 2. She won OTFA's 1500m, placed 2nd in her age category at the 2004 Ironman Canada (10:38:06) and achieved a personal best at the 2013 Scotia Bank Toronto Waterfront Half Marathon (1:21:43).

Sharlene Cobain is a runner and mother of 2. She achieved personal bests at the 2007 Toronto Half Marathon (1:20:56) and 2007 Mississauga Marathon (2:54:39) and frequently places within the top 10.

Stephanie Hewitt is a squash player and mother of 3. She is a 3-time World Women's Open Squash Doubles Champion, ranked in the top 3 in the world in women's professional doubles since 2006, and ranked 1st in the Canadian Women's Doubles Squash.

Stephanie Summers is a triathlete, runner and mother of 2. She received a full scholarship to a U.S. university and participated twice at the World's Triathlon Championship.

Susie Mitchell is a track cyclist and mother of 1. She won a gold medal at the 2012 World Track Master's Championship in the individual pursuit, won 2 silver medals at the 2013 World Track Master's Championship and has 5 Irish National Championship titles in track cycling. Her book, *Pregnancy to Podium* speaks about her training during pregnancy and regaining peak fitness post birth.

Tania Jones is a marathoner runner and mother of 2. She was the 2002 Canadian Marathon female Champion, placed 44th in the 2001 World Track and Field Marathon Championship and holds the Canadian record for the indoor 4X800m event.

Tara Norton is a professional triathlete and mother of 1. She placed 12th at the 2007 Ford Ironman World Championship, placed 2nd at the 2007 Ironman Lanzarote and holds the bike course record at Ironman Lanzarote.

Wendy Simms is a cyclist and mother of 2. She is a 5-time National Cyclocross Champion, a top 10 finisher at Cyclocross World Championship and a Canadian National team member for mountain biking and cyclocross.

Zoe Webster is a runner, mountain biker and mother of 2. Her personal best for a marathon is 3:13:05 and 1:34:25 for a half marathon. She ran the Boston Marathon and is one of the models in our book.

Our Professionals

Adrienne McRuvie is a chiropractor, acupuncturist, yoga therapist and a HypnoBirthing doula. Adrienne graduated from the Canadian Memorial Chiropractic College and received her doula training from DONA. She currently runs a wellness family practice in the east end of Toronto. www.omachiro.com

Alexis Williams is a registered dietician and is currently Senior Director Wellness at Loblaw Companies Limited. She was awarded a BSc and MSc in Applied Nutrition from the University of Guelph. She also has a diploma in Sport Nutrition from the International Olympic Committee. She has written for Running Room magazine and is an avid triathlete. She is the proud mother of 1.

Andrea Page is a certified personal trainer, sport strength specialist and childbirth-trained educator. In 2000 she founded and became CEO of Andrea Page's Original Fitmom and currently offers Andrea Page's Original Fitmom programs in 8 different cities across North America via the Andrea Page's Original Fitmom Licensing and Certification program. www.fitmomfitness.com

Angela Dufour has worked as a dietitian within the health and fitness and food service industries since 1999. She holds Bachelor of Science in Human Ecology and Master's degree in Adult Education (MEd) both from Mount Saint Vincent University. In 2007, Angela graduated with the International Olympic Committee's Graduate Sports Nutrition Diploma. She is also a level 1 ISAK anthropometrist. She is an avid runner and proud mother of 1 little boy. www.nutritioninaction.ca

Anna Maria Infante graduated as a chiropodist from the Michener Institute in 1998. She has worked as a clinical instructor for the Michener Institute and has served on the Board of Directors of the Ontario Society of Chiropodists. Since 1998 she has owned and operated Family Foot Care in Bolton and Orangeville. www.familyfootcare.net

Christine Matheson is a naturopathic doctor who completed her training at the Canadian College of Naturopathic Medicine in 2001. She is respected for her pioneering role in the field as one of the first naturopathic doctor's in Canada to work in a hospital setting as a member of an integrative medical team of doctors and specialists at the former Women's Pelvic Health Centre at Women's College Hospital in Toronto. Christine is recognized particularly for her specific clinical experience in women's health, pelvic health, gynecology, urology, pre and post natal care and children's health. Christine is currently in private practice in 2 well-established clinics in downtown Toronto. www.christinemathesonnd.com

Clifford Librach is a board certified fertility specialist. He is an Associate Professor at the University of Toronto Department of Obstetrics and Gynecology and chief of the division of Reproductive Biology at the Sunnybrook Health Sciences Centre and the Women's College Hospital in Toronto. He is also the founder and director of the Create Fertility Centre in Toronto. Dr. Librach directs a large research program and has authored numerous research publications in the fertility field. Dr. Librach is frequently interviewed on television, radio and print and has served on several national committees related to reproductive technologies.

Dallas Parsons is an International Board Certified Lactation Consultant and dietitian. She earned her Diploma in Lactation Medicine from the International Breast Clinic. Dallas has over 3000 hours working with mom and babies. She started her dietetics career in the area of sports medicine and has worked with numerous athletes including Canada's top Olympians. She is the proud mother of 3. www.beststartlc.com

Dragana Boljanovic-Susic is a graduate of McMaster University, with Master's degree in Rehabilitation Sciences. She is an experienced physiotherapist and has been long interested in the treatment of women's health concerns and chronic and neuropathic pain in individuals with musculoskeletal issues. She has been an invited lecturer and a clinical instructor at the University of Toronto since 2003. She played a significant role in Women's Health Pelvic Centre at Women's College Hospital as their only physiotherapist.

Hasinah Shaqiq has an Advanced Diploma in Podiatric Medicine with Distinction (D.Pod.M) from the Michener Institute. Her practical training includes 3 years of combined clinical and theory experience at St. John's Rehabilitation, the Toronto Rehabilitation Hospital, Sherbourne Health Centre and Women's College Hospital. She currently works at MedCan Clinic. www.medcan.com/medcan_team/hasinah_shaqiq/

Jennifer Sygo is a dietitian who holds a degree in Biochemistry from McMaster University and Nutritional Sciences from the University of Guelph. Jennifer is in private practice at Cleveland Clinic Canada and is a leading sports nutritionist for the Coaching Association of Canada. She has worked with all types of athletes; from recreational level to Olympic and world medalists, as well as professional athletes and is currently the dietitian for Canada's national track and field team. Jennifer is also an author and is regularly featured in the television and print media. www.jennifersygo.com

Jennifer Wise is a chiropractor who received a Bachelor of Health Sciences degree from the University of Western Ontario and completed her chiropractic studies at Life University in Atlanta Georgia. She did her perinatal and pediatric chiropractic training through the International Chiropractic Pediatric Association. www.thrivehealth.ca

Jenny Hadfield is a running and fitness expert, an author and adventure-preneur who inspires every day mortals to run their best lives and earn beautiful views. Jenny has a Bachelor's degree in Education and Health Promotion and a Master's degree in Exercise Science. Jenny has published two books, *"Running for Mortals"* and *"Marathoning for Mortals"*. She has a weekly column on RunnersWorld.com, her monthly column in Women's Running Magazine and has been featured in numerous media outlets such as Women's Health, The Chicago Tribune, and Good Morning America – Health. Jenny has competed in running and adventure races all over the world. www.jennyhadfield.com

Jon Barrett is the head of the maternal-fetal medicine program at Sunnybrook Health Sciences Centre. Dr. Barrett is also an Associate Scientist for Evaluative Clinical Sciences, Women & Babies Research Program (Director) for Sunnybrook Research Institute (SRI) and Associate Professor in the Department of Obstetrics and Gynaecology at the University of Toronto. In addition to providing general prenatal and obstetrical care, he also specializes in the care of women with high-risk twin/multiple pregnancies. www.sunnybrook.ca/research/team/member. asp?t=10&m=21&page=191

Julia Alleyne is a Family Physician practicing Sport and Exercise Medicine at the Toronto Rehabilitation Institute, University Health Network. In addition, she trained as a physiotherapist and maintained an active license for 30 years. She is appointed at the University of Toronto, Department of Family and Community Medicine as an associate clinical professor. Dr. Alleyne is the past-President of the Canadian Academy of Sport Medicine and the Chief Medical Office for the 2015 Pan and Parapan American Games in Toronto. She was selected to the 2002, 2006, 2008 and 2010 Olympic Medical Staff and served as the Chief Medical Office for the Canadian team for the 2012 Summer Olympics. Her research and educational programs have been focused on Women and Sport and she was honoured by the Canadian Association for the Advancement of Women in Sport and Physical Activity as a recipient of the 2003 Most Influential Women in Sport and Physical Activity Award. www.drjulia.net

Julie Toole is a registered midwife with a BHSc from the Midwifery Education Program at Ryerson University and a Master of Science degree in Medical Sciences from the Joint Centre for Bioethics at the University of Toronto. She currently works as a risk management specialist at the Association of Ontario Midwives. Julie is also an adjunct Assistant Professor at the Schulich Interfaculty Program in Public Health at Western University and is an instructor at WattsUp cycling. Julie is an avid cyclist, sometimes bike racer and mother to 2 wonderfully active little girls. Follow Julie's ramblings on twitter @julie_toole

Kevin Jardine is a chiropractor, health and fitness expert, entrepreneur and innovator in the field of physical and rehabilitative medicine. He graduated from the Canadian Memorial Chiropractic College and is owner of a multidisciplinary sports therapy clinic in Toronto called The Urban Athlete. He treats and advises numerous professional and Olympic athletes and teams. As an entrepreneur, Dr. Jardine was a co-creator of SpiderTech products and education, president and co-owner of Collaborans and founder of FPR. He is also a speaker and writer who has the unique ability take complex information and transform it into understandable clinical insight. www.theurbanathlete.ca

Lianne Phillipson-Webb is a registered nutritionist who graduated from Institute of Optimum Nutrition in London, England. She is founder of Sprout Right, a company that specializes in pre-conception, prenatal, and postnatal nutrition for women as well as good nutrition for the whole family. Since graduating, she shares her knowledge with thousands of women and their families through personal consultations, television appearances, contributions in magazines and online parenting websites, interactive workshops, one-of-a-kind Mommy Chef cooking classes and her company's instructional DVD series. www.sproutright.com

Michelle Mottola is the Director of R. Samuel McLaughlin Foundation Exercise and Pregnancy Laboratory at Western University, the only lab in North America that specializes in the area of exercising pregnant and post-partum women. For over 20 years Dr. Mottola, an anatomist and exercise physiologist, has conducted research on the effects of maternal exercise on both the mother and the developing fetus. She has authored numerous peer-reviewed articles, presented her research at conferences worldwide and has been featured in many media outlets including television, newspapers and magazines. www.uwo.ca/fhs/EPL

Moira Merrithew, following a successful career as a principal ballet dancer, went on to retrain and certify as a Pilates instructor. Along with husband Lindsay G. Merrithew, the pair co-founded Merrithew Health & Fitness™ where they have worked for over 25 years to develop programs that promote the benefits of responsible exercise and mindful movement, such as STOTT PILATES®, ZEN•GA™, CORE™ Athletic Conditioning & Performance Training™ and Total Barre™. Together, they work with a team of physical therapists, sports medicine and fitness professionals to ensure that all programming is aligned with the latest finding in biomechanical research and exercise science. Moira is also the Executive Director of Education and oversees the creation of curricula and support materials. www.merrithew.com

Monica Voss has been studying and teaching yoga for over 35 years. She practiced and taught yoga during all her pregnancies and while raising her 3 children. She is co-owner and director of the Esther Myer studio in Toronto. In addition to teaching classes at the studio, Monica conducts workshops, retreats and teacher training internationally. www. estheryoga.com

Natalie Wright graduated from the Midwifery Education Program at Ryerson University in 2005. Prior to becoming a midwife, Natalie was an early childhood educator and doula. She has worked in various communities throughout Great Britain and Canada. www. allistonmidwives.ca

Nicole Stevenson is one of Canada's top elite runners and has been racing for over 25 years. She has competed all types of races from 5k to marathons. She is a performance running coach and is a regular columnist with Canadian Running. She currently coaches the Angels, an elite and developmental team of female runners. www.runwithspr.com

Pam Ennis is a manual osteopathic practitioner who graduated from the Canadian College of Osteopathy in 2008. Prior to becoming an osteopath, Pam received a Bachelor's degree in Physical Education from the University of Toronto in 1995. She combines both of her specialties in her practice to ensure optimal health of her clients. Pam also specializes in women's issues and pediatrics. www.pamennis.com

Tara Postnikoff is a registered nutritional consulting practitioner, triathlon coach and personal trainer who holds an Honours Bachelor degree in Anthropology (and minor in Biology) from McMaster University. In 2006, Tara established HEAL (Healthy Eating Active Living). She is a writer for Running Room magazine and has contributed to Canadian Cycling and Triathlon Canada magazines. www.heal-nutrition.com

Taya Griffin is a breastfeeding consultant with over 700 hours of clinical experience helping mothers reach their breastfeeding goals. In 2007, Taya graduated from Ontario College of Homeopathic Medicine in Health Sciences and Homeopathic Medicine and in 2011 from the International Breastfeeding Centre/Newman Breastfeeding Clinic's Lactation Medicine Program. In addition, she is on the faculty of the Ontario College of Homeopathic Medicine teaching about homeopathy, pregnancy, labour and breastfeeding. She also teaches yoga and Pilates to pre and postnatal mothers. www.tayagriffin.com

Trish Del Sorbo, a business expert in the fitness industry, has managed, owned and taught in profitable fitness clubs and pre/post-natal care facilities in Canada and Europe over the last twenty years. Trish was owner and director of Toronto's Baby and Me Fitness, North America's original pre/postnatal fitness company from 2006 -2013.

GLOSSARY

GLOSSARY

Abscesses: Painful areas of inflamed tissue that are filled with pus.

Abdominal Aorta: The large artery that supplies oxygenated blood to all of the abdominal and pelvic organs, as well as the legs.

Absolute Contraindications: Threatening conditions or factors that warrant discontinuing exercise.

Active Release Treatment: A soft tissue method commonly used to treat conditions related to adhesions or scar tissue in overused muscles.

Adverse Effects: Harmful and undesired effects resulting from a medication or other intervention.

Amenorrhea: The absence of menstruation and ovulation.

Anemia: A condition marked by a deficiency of red blood cells or haemoglobin in the blood.

Anovulation: Regular cycles with failure to develop and release an egg (lack of ovulation).

APGAR Scores: A measure of the physical condition of a newborn infant. Measures include: appearance (skin colour), pulse rate (heart rate), grimace response (reflexes), activity (muscle tone) and respiration (breathing rate and effort).

Blood Clots: Collection of sticky blood cells that form in response to damage of a blood vessel.

Blood Volume: The total amount of blood in the body.

Body Mass Index (BMI): A number calculated using a person's weight and height. It is a fairly reliable indicator of body fat for most people. It is calculated using the person's weight in kilograms (kg) divided by his or her height in metres squared (BMI=weight (kg)/ height (m)^2).

Blood Glucose: The amount of glucose in the blood; glucose is the main sugar that the body makes from food in the diet and provides energy to all cells in the body.

Cardiovascular System: A system that consists of the heart and blood vessels that circulates blood throughout the body.

Carpel Tunnel Syndrome: A painful wrist condition that occurs when the median nerve, which runs from the forearm into the palm of the hand, becomes compressed or squeezed at the wrist.

Case Study: A type of observational data collection technique in which a single person is studied to identify behavioural, emotional and/or cognitive qualities that may be applicable to others.

Centre of Gravity: The place in your body where your weight is evenly dispersed and all sides are in balance.

Core Strength: The balanced development of the deep and superficial muscles that stabilize, align and move the trunk of the body. It goes beyond the surface muscles and utilizes the deep internal muscles to maintain stability in motion. Also referred to as *core stability*.

Diabetes: A medical condition in which a person has high blood sugar, either because the body does not produce enough insulin or because cells do not respond to the insulin that is produced.

Diastasis Recti: A condition where the connective tissue (linea alba) connecting the 2 halves of the abdominal muscles along the midline of the torso stretches and separates.

Dyspnea: Shortness of breath.

Episiotomy: A surgical cut between the vagina and anus.

Exercising: A term used to describe one's intention to workout in a less-scheduled manner and with no concrete goal or expectation.

Exercise Duration: The amount of time that a person exercises for.

Exercising Heart Rate: Refers to the number of times your heart beats over the course of 1 minute during a bout of exercise.

Exercise Intensity: The level of effort or exertion that a person executes while exercising.

Exercise Volume: The amount or quantity that a person exercises during a given period of time.

Extension: The range of motion that increases a joint angle. For example, moving from a sitting position to standing position allows you to extend your hip and knee joints.

Fartleks: A Swedish word meaning "speed play" that refers to a training technique consisting of bursts of more intense effort alternating with less intense, strenuous activity.

Fetal Abnormalities: An abnormal condition in a fetus.

Fetus: A developing human from usually 2 months after conception to birth.

Flexion: The range of motion that decreases a joint angle; bending. For example, lifting your coffee cup to your mouth flexes your elbow joint.

Follicle Stimulating Hormone (FSH): Is a hormone that helps to control the menstrual cycle and the production of eggs by the ovaries. There is an increase in this hormone just before the egg is released (ovulation).

Gestational Age: The period of time between conception and birth during which the fetus grows and develops inside the mother's womb.

Gestational Diabetes: Any degree of glucose intolerance with onset or first recognition during pregnancy.

Graston Technique: An instrument-assisted soft tissue technique.

Hypertension: High blood pressure.

Incompetent Cervix: Uterine cervix dilates before term and without labour, possibly resulting in miscarriage or premature birth.

Incontinence: The inability to control urination.

Infertility: Diminished or absent ability to conceive and have children.

Joint Laxity: Lack of stability in the joint; can be induced by pregnancy.

Kyphosis: The outward or bowing curvature of the thoracic (mid-back) spine.

Lactic Acid: A naturally occurring by-product that builds up in your muscles and blood during strenuous exercise.

Lateral Flexion: Movement of the head, trunk and/or limbs away from the midline and out to the side.

Luteinizing Hormone (LH): A hormone that helps to regulate the menstrual cycle and egg production. It increases just before ovulation, around the middle of the cycle (i.e. day 14 of a 28 day cycle).

Lordosis: The inward curvature of the lumbar (low back) and cervical (neck) spine.

Meta-Analysis: A statistical technique used to summarize the results of experimental studies that address a common problem.

Obstetric Complications: Deviations from an expected, normal course of events or offspring development during pregnancy, labour-delivery and the early neonatal period.

Organ prolapse: The muscles and ligaments supporting a woman's pelvic organs weaken or stretch from childbirth or surgery and as a result, the pelvic organs may slip out of place (prolapse). Common types of prolapse include urethra, bladder, uterus, small bowel or rectum.

Osteopathy: A philosophy and type of practice that emphasizes the interrelationship between structure and function of the body and recognizes the body's ability to heal itself.

Ovulation: The release of an egg from the ovary; this must happen in order to achieve pregnancy.

Pelvic Stability: The ability of the body's trunk and hip/pelvic muscles to keep the spine and pelvis in optimal alignment during activity.

Perineum: The area between the vagina and anus.

Placenta: A temporary organ that joins the mother and fetus, transferring oxygen and nutrients from the mother to the fetus and permitting the release of carbon dioxide and waste products from the fetus.

Placenta Previa: A condition in which the placenta is abnormally placed and partially or totally covers the cervix.

Postpartum: Period after giving birth; whereas some will classify it as the period immediately following childbirth up until 6 weeks, others will not limit the duration period. Can be used interchangeably with "postnatal".

Pre-Conception: The period occurring prior to conception or conceiving.

Preeclampsia: High blood pressure and excess protein in the urine after 20 weeks of pregnancy in a woman with previously normal blood pressure. Left untreated, preeclampsia can lead to serious complications for mother and baby.

Premature Labour or Preterm Birth or Preterm Delivery: The birth of a baby at less than 37 weeks gestational age.

Presyncope: A state consisting of light-headedness, muscular weakness and feeling faint.

Pronation: A slight inward rolling motion of the foot during normal walking or running stride. "Normal" pronation is when the foot rolls inward approximately 15%. Greater than that is called "over-pronation".

Randomized Control Trial (RCT): A quantitative, comparative, controlled experiment in which people are allocated at random (by chance) to receive 1 of several interventions, including the standard intervention (known as control group). This type of study seeks to measure and compare the outcomes of the intervention following completion of the study. RCTs are one of the simplest and most powerful tools in clinical research.

Rate of Perceived Exertion: A method to determine exercise intensity; uses a scale of 6-20 to rate effort level.

Range of Motion: The total range through which a joint can be moved.

Relative Contraindications: Less threatening conditions or factors but still dangerous enough warranting supervision and modifications to exercise.

Relaxin: A hormone produced during pregnancy that facilitates the birth process by causing a softening and lengthening of the cervix and the pubic symphysis (the place where the pubic bones come together). It is also responsible for joint laxity in the entire body during this time.

Respiratory System: Comprised of the organs in your body that help you to breathe; gas exchange occurs here allowing oxygen to be delivered to the body and carbon dioxide (waste) to be taken away.

Resting Heart Rate: Refers to the number of times your heart beats in a single minute while at rest.

Rotation: The range of motion that refers to movement toward or away from the midline of the body. For example, turning your head to the right or left without moving your body.

Ruptured Membranes: The rupture of the amniotic sac.

Sacroiliac Joint: Located on either side of the low back at the point where the 2 hip bones (ilium) meet the sacrum (tailbone). The joint is held in place by a number of strong ligaments. Also referred to as the "SI joint".

Spontaneous Abortion: The unplanned loss of pregnancy.

Superior Vena Cava: The large vein that returns blood to the heart from the head, neck and both upper limbs.

Supine Position: Lying on one's back.

Talk Test: A method used to determine exercise intensity; a comfortable intensity is when a person is able to maintain a conversation during exercise.

Tempo: A training technique where cardiovascular activity is performed at a steady effort level.

Thyroid Disease: A medical condition impairing the function of the thyroid.

Training: A term used to describe one's commitment to some form of a plan that enables her to work toward a specific goal and may include a larger volume and/or more intense activity.

Uterine Growth Restriction: Inadequate fetal growth during pregnancy.

Varicose Veins: Veins that have become enlarged and twisted.

HELPFUL RESOURCES

HELPFUL RESOURCES

DESCRIPTION	LINK OR CONTACT
American College of Obstetricians and Gynecologists (ACOG)	
With close to 55,000 members, ACOG strongly advocates for quality health care for women, maintains the highest standards of clinical practice and continuing education of its members, promotes patient education and increases awareness among its members and the public of the changing issues facing women's health care.	Main website: www.acog.org Committee opinion on Exercise and Pregnancy: www.acog.org/Resources-And-Publications/Committee-Opinions/Committee-on-Obstetric-Practice/Exercise-During-Pregnancy-and-the-Postpartum-Period
American College of Sports Medicine (ACSM)	
ACSM is the largest sports medicine and exercise science organization in the world. It works to advance and integrate scientific research to provide educational and practical applications of exercise science and sports medicine.	Main website: www.acsm.org Pregnancy-related information: www.acsm.org/search-results?q=exercise%20and%20pregnancy
American Pregnancy Association	
American Pregnancy Association is a national health organization committed to promoting reproductive and pregnancy wellness through education, support, advocacy and community awareness.	Main website: www.americanpregnancy.org
Canadian Academy of Sport and Exercise Medicine (CASEM)	
CASEM is an organization of physicians committed to excellence in the practice of medicine as it applies to all aspects of physical activity.	Main website: www.casem-acmse.org Pregnancy-related information: www.casem-acmse.org/education/position-statements/

Canadian Society for Exercise Physiology (CSEP)	
CSEP is the principal body for physical activity, health and fitness research and personal training in Canada.	Main website: www.csep.ca Pregnancy-related information (PARmed-X for Pregnancy): www.csep.ca/cmfiles/publications/parq/parmed-xpreg.pdf
Exercise and Pregnancy Help Line	
A toll-free helpline in North America providing free information relating to exercise during pregnancy. The helpline is affiliated with Women's College Hospital and Mother Risk at the Hospital for Sick Children in Toronto, Ontario.	1.866.937.7678
Health Canada	
Health Canada is the Federal department responsible for helping Canadians maintain and improve their health, while respecting individual choices and circumstances.	Main web site: www.hc-sc.gc.ca Healthy Weight Gain During Pregnancy: www.hc-sc.gc.ca/fn-an/nutrition/prenatal/hwgdp-ppspg-eng.php
Society Obstetricians and Gynaecologists of Canada (SOGC)	
SOGC is a national medical society in Canada, representing over 3,000 obstetricians, gynecologists, family physicians, nurses, midwives and allied health professionals in the field of sexual reproductive health. It promotes excellence in the practice of obstetrics and works to advance the health of women through leadership, advocacy, collaboration, outreach and education.	Main web site: www.sogc.org Pregnancy-related information: www.pregnancy.sogc.org

REFERENCES

REFERENCES

REFERENCES

THE GAME PLAN

Hammer RL, Perkins J, Parr R. Exercise during the childbearing year. The Journal of Perinatal Education. 2000; 9(1): 1-13.

PREPARING YOUR BODY FOR PREGNANCY

Chapter 1: Training for Conception
American College of Sports Medicine. [Internet]. Indianapolis: ASCM Current Comment. Menstrual Cycle Dysfunction; c unknown [last modified unknown; cited June 2012]; [about 3 screens]. Available from: https://www.acsm.org/docs/current-comments/menstrualcycledysfunction.pdf

American Society of Reproductive Medicine [Internet]. Birmingham: American Society for Reproductive Medicine. Infertility. ©1996-2014 [last modified unknown; cited 15 May 2009]; [about 1 screen]. Available from: http://www.reproductivefacts.org/awards/detail.aspx?id=10707

Clapp, JF III. Exercising through your pregnancy. Omaha: Atticus Books; 2002.

Homan G, Litt J, Norman RJ. The FAST study: Fertility assessment and advice targeting lifestyle choices and behaviours: a pilot study. Human Reproduction. 2012;37(8):2396-404.

Marquez S, Molinero O. Energy availability, menstrual dysfunction and bone health in sports; an overview of the female athlete triad. Nutricion Hospitalaria. 2013;28(4):1010-17.

Minster of Public Works and Government Services Canada [Internet]. Ottawa: Health Canada. Body Mass Index (BMI) Nomogram; c2003[last modified 2012 Feb 23; cited 23 June 2013]; [about 1 screen]. Available from: http://www.hc-sc.gc.ca/fn-an/nutrition/weights-poids/guide-ld-adult/bmi_chart_java-graph_imc_java-eng.php

Nattiv A, Loucks AB, Manore MM, Sanborn CR, Sundgot-Borgen J, Warren MP. American College of Sports Medicine Position stand: The female triad. Medicine & Science in Sports & Exercise. 2007;39(10):1867-82.

New York Times [Internet]. New York: New York Times Magazine. Bodies at work: Six variations on the Olympic Ideal; cJuly 2008 [last modified unknown; cited May 2013]; [about 7 screens]. Available from: http://www.nytimes.com/slideshow/2008/07/30/magazine/803BODIES_2.html?_r=0

Olive DL. Exercise and fertility: an update. Current Opinion in Obstetrics and Gynecology. 2010;22(4):259-63.

Redman LM, Loucks AB. Menstrual disorders in athletes. Sports Medicine. 2005;35(9):747-55.

Roupas ND, Georgopoulos NA. Menstrual function in sports. Hormones. 2011;10(2):104-16.

Warren MP, Perlroth NE. Hormones and sport: The effects of intense exercise on the female reproductive system. Journal of Endocrinology. 2001;170:3-11.

Chapter 2: Getting Yourself to the Start Line

Brumitt J. A return to running program for the postpartum client: A case report. Physiotherapy Theory and Practice. 2009;25(4):310-25.

Hale RW, Milne L. The elite athlete and exercise in pregnancy. Seminars in Perinatology. 1996;29(4):277-84.

Moore KL, Dalley AF. Clinically oriented anatomy, fourth edition. Philadelphia: Lippincot, Williams & Wilkins; 1999.

TRAINING FOR TWO

Chapter 3: The Pregnant Athlete's Body

American Pregnancy Association [Internet]. Texas: American Pregnancy Association. Eating for two when over/or under weight; c2012[last modified 2014 June; cited June 2013]; [about 1 screen]. Available from: http://americanpregnancy.org/pregnancyhealth/aboutpregweightgain.html

Artal R, O'Toole M. Guidelines of the American College of Obstetricians and Gynecologists for exercise during pregnancy and the postpartum period. British Journal of Sports Medicine. 2003;37(1):6-12.

Gryedanus DE, Patel DR. The female athlete before and beyond puberty. The Pediatric Clinics of North America. 2002;49:553-80.

Hammer RL, Perkins J, Parr R. Exercise during the childbearing year. The Journal of Perinatal Education. 2000; 9(1):1-13.

Health Canada [Internet]. Ottawa: Health Canada. Weight gain during pregnancy: Re-examining the guidelines; c2010 [last modified 2010 Nov 08; cited 23 June 2013]; [about 1 screen]. Available from: http://www.hc-sc.gc.ca/fn-an/nutrition/prenatal/ewba-mbsa-eng.php#t3

Kawaguchi JK and Pickering RK. The pregnant athlete, part 1: Anatomy and physiology of pregnancy. Athletic Therapy Today. 2010;15(2):39-43.

Chapter 4: Exercise and Pregnancy 101

American College of Sports Medicine. Exercise prescription for healthy populations and special considerations. In: ACSMs Guidelines for Exercise Testing and Prescription, Eighth Edition. Philadephia: Wolters Kluwer and Lippincott Williams & Wilkins; 2013. p. 183-7.

ACOG Committee on Obstetric Practice [Internet]. Washington: The American Congress of Obstetricians and Gynecologists. Number 267 Exercise during pregnancy and the postpartum period. c2002; [last modified unknown; cited August 2009]; [about 1 page]. Available from: http://www.acog.org/Resources-And-Publications/Committee-Opinions/Committee-on-Obstetric-Practice/Exercise-During-Pregnancy-and-the-Postpartum-Period

Alleyne J, Peticca P. Canadian Academy of Sport and Exercise Medicine [Internet]. Ottawa: Canadian Academy of Sport and Exercise Medicine. Exercise and Pregnancy Position Statement and Discussion Paper; c2008 [last modified unknown; cited August 2009]; [about 18 pages]. Available from: http://casem-acmse.org/wp-content/uploads/2013/07/Discussion-Paper-Pregnancy.pdf

The American College of Obstetricians and Gynecologists [Internet]. Washington: The American Congress of Obstetricians and Gynecologists. Frequently asked questions during pregnancy. c2011; [last modified unknown; cited March 2013]; [about 1 page]. Available from: http://www.acog.org/Patients/FAQs/Exercise-During-Pregnancy

Canadian Academy of Sport and Exercise Medicine Sport Safety [Internet]. Ottawa: Committee Canadian Academy of Sport and Exercise Medicine. Position statement. Exercise and pregnancy; c2008 [last modified unknown; cited August 2009]; [about 3 pages]. Available from: http://casem-acmse.org/wp-content/uploads/2013/07/Exercise-Pregnancy-Position-Paper-_2008_.pdf

Bauer PW, Broman CL, Pivarnik JM. Exercise and pregnancy knowledge among healthcare providers. Journal of Women's Health. 2010; 19(2):335-41.

Davies GA, Wolfe LA, Mottola MF, MacKinnon C. Joint SOGC/CSEP clinical practice guideline: exercise in pregnancy and the postpartum period. Canadian Journal of Applied Physiology. 2003;28(3):330-41.

Evenson KR, Barakat R, Brown WJ, Dargent-Molina P, Haruna M, Mikkelsen EM, Mottola MF, Owe KM, Rousham EK, Yeo S. Guidelines for physical activity during pregnancy: Comparisons from around the world. American Journal of Lifestyle Medicine. 2014;8(2):102-21.

Hammer RL, Perkins J, Parr R. Exercise during the childbearing years. The Journal of Perinatal Education. 2000;9(1):1-13.

Jefferys R. The pregnant exerciser: An argument for exercise as a means to support pregnancy. ACSM's Certified News. 2005;15(3):5-7.

Labonte-Lemoyne Curnier Ellemberg. Foetal brain development is influenced by maternal exercise during pregnancy. Program No. 217.08. 2013 Neuroscience Meeting Planner. San Deigo, CA: Society for Neuroscience. 2013, Online.

Mottola MF. Exercise prescription for overweight and obese women: Pregnancy and postpartum. Obstetrics & Gynecology Clinics of North America. 2009;36:301-16.

Wolfe LA, Mottola MF. Canadian Society for Exercise Physiology [Internet]. Ottawa: Canadian Society for Exercise Physiology. Physical Activity Readiness Medical Examination for Pregnancy. c1999;[last modified 2013; cited Aug 2009]; [about 4 pages]. Available from: http://www.csep.ca/cmfiles/publications/parq/parmed-xpreg.pdf

Chapter 5: To Train or Not To Train?
ACOG Committee on Obstetric Practice [Internet]. Washington: The American Congress of Obstetricians and Gynecologists. Number 267 Exercise during pregnancy and the postpartum period. c2002; [last modified unknown; cited August 2009]; [about 1 page]. Available from: http://www.acog.org/Resources-And-Publications/Committee-Opinions/Committee-on-Obstetric-Practice/Exercise-During-Pregnancy-and-the-Postpartum-Period

American College of Sports Medicine. Exercise prescription for healthy populations and special considerations. In: ACSMs Guidelines for Exercise Testing and Prescription, Eighth Edition. Philadephia: Wolters Kluwer and Lippincott Williams & Wilkins; 2013. p. 183-7.

Davies GA, Wolfe LA, Mottola MF, MacKinnon C. Joint SOGC/CSEP clinical practice guideline: exercise in pregnancy and the postpartum period. Canadian Journal of Applied Physiology. 2003;28(3):330-41.

Hammer RL, Perkins J, Parr R. Exercise during the childbearing year. The Journal of Perinatal Education. 2000;9(1):1-13.

Wolfe LA, Mottola MF. Canadian Society for Exercise Physiology [Internet]. Ottawa: Canadian Society for Exercise Physiology. Physical Activity Readiness Medical Examination for Pregnancy. c1999;[last modified 2013; cited Aug 2009]; [about 4 pages]. Available from: http://www.csep.ca/cmfiles/publications/parq/parmed-xpreg.pdf

Chapter 6: How Hard, How Often and How Long?
ACOG Committee on Obstetric Practice [Internet]. Washington: The American Congress of Obstetricians and Gynecologists. Number 267 Exercise during pregnancy and the postpartum period. c2002; [last modified unknown; cited August 2009]; [about 1 page]. Available from: http://www.acog.org/Resources-And-Publications/Committee-Opinions/Committee-on-Obstetric-Practice/Exercise-During-Pregnancy-and-the-Postpartum-Period

Alleyne J, Peticca P. Canadian Academy of Sport and Exercise Medicine [Internet]. Ottawa: Canadian Academy of Sport and Exercise Medicine. Exercise and Pregnancy Position Statement and Discussion Paper; c2008 [last modified unknown; cited August 2009]; [about

18 pages]. Available from: http://casem-acmse.org/wp-content/uploads/2013/07/Discussion-Paper-Pregnancy.pdf

American College of Sports Medicine. Exercise prescription for healthy populations and special considerations. In: ACSMs Guidelines for Exercise Testing and Prescription, Eighth Edition. Philadephia: Lippincott Williams & Wilkins; 2013. p. 183-7.

Bell, R. The effects of vigorous exercise during pregnancy on birth weight. Journal of Science and Medicine in Sport. 2002;5(1):32-6.

Bell RJ, Palma SM, Lumley JM. The effects of vigorous exercise during pregnancy on birth-weight. Australian and New Zealand Journal of Obstetrics and Gynaecology. 1995;35(1):46-51.

Campbell MK, Mottola MF. Recreational exercise and occupational activity during pregnancy and birth weight: A case-control study. American Journal of Obstetrics and Gynecology. 2001:184(3):403-8.

Chasan-Taber L, Evenson KR, Sternfeld B, Kengeri S. Assessment of recreational activity during pregnancy in epidemiologic studies of birthweight and length of gestation: methodologic aspects. Women & Health. 2007;45(4):85-107.

Canadian Academy of Sport and Exercise Medicine Sport Safety Committee [Internet]. Canadian Academy of Sport and Exercise Medicine. Ottawa: Canadian Academy of Sport and Exercise Medicine. Position statement. Exercise and pregnancy; c2008 [last modified unknown; cited August 2009]; [about 3 pages]. Available from: http://casem-acmse.org/wp-content/uploads/2013/07/Exercise-Pregnancy-Position-Paper-_2008_.pdf

Clapp, JF III. Exercising through your pregnancy. Omaha: Atticus Books; 2002.

Davenport MH, Charlesworth S, Vanderspank D, Sopper MM, Mottola MF. Development and validation of exercise target heart rate zones for overweight and obese pregnant women. Applied Physiology, Nutrition, and Metabolism. 2008;33:984-9.

Davies GA, Wolfe LA, Mottola MF, MacKinnon C. Joint SOGC/CSEP clinical practice guideline: exercise in pregnancy and the postpartum period. Canadian Journal of Applied Physiology. 2003;28(3):330-41.

Duncombe D, Skouteris H, Wertheim EH, Kelly L, Fraser V, Paxton SJ. Vigorous exercise and birth outcomes in a sample of recreational exercisers: A prospective study across pregnancy. Australian and New Zealand Journal of Obstetrics and Gynaecology. 2006;46(4):288-92.

Evenson KR, Moos MK, Carrier K, Siega-Riz AM. Perceived barriers to physical activity among pregnant women. Maternal and Child Health Journal. 2009;13(3):364-75.

Evenson KR, Siega-Riz AM, Savitz DA, Leiferman JA, Thorp JM. Vigorous leisure activity and pregnancy outcome. Epidemiology. 2002;13(6):653-9.

Hale RW, Milne L. The elite athlete and exercise in pregnancy. Seminars in Perinatology. 1996;29(4):277-84.

Hatch MC, Shu XO, McLean DE, Levin B, Begg M, Reuss L, Susser M. Maternal exercise during pregnancy, physical fitness and fetal growth. American Journal of Epidemiology. 1993; 137(10):1105-14.

Kawaguchi JK and Pickering RK. The pregnant athlete, part 2: Exercise recommendations. Athletic Therapy Today, 2010;15(3):38-41.

Kardel KR. Effects of intense training during and after pregnancy in top-level athletes. Scandinavian Journal of Medicine & Science in Sports. 2005;15:79-86.

Kardel KR, Kase T. Training in pregnant women: Effects of fetal development and birth. American Journal of Obstetrics and Gynecology. 1998;178(2):280-6.

Kramer MS and McDonald SW. Aerobic exercise for women during pregnancy. Cochrane Database of Systematic Reviews 2006, Issue 3. Art. No.: CD000180. DOI: 10.1002/14651858. CD000180.pub2

Leet T, Flick L. Effects of exercise on birthweight. Clinical Obstetrics and Gynecology. 2003;46(2):423-31.

Lockey EA, Tran ZV, Wells CL, Myers BC, Tran AC. Effects of physical exercise on pregnancy outcomes: a meta-analytic review. Medicine & Science in Sports & Exercise. 1991;23(11):1234-9.

Mottola FM, Inglis S, Brun CR, Hammond JR. Physiological and metabolic responses of late pregnant women to 40 minutes of steady-state exercise followed by an oral glucose tolerance perturbation. Journal of Applied Physiology. 2013;115(5):597-604.

Mottola MF. Exercise and pregnancy: Canadian guidelines for health care professionals. Alberta Centre for Active Living: Well Spring. 2011;22(4).

Mottola MF. Exercise prescription for overweight and obese women: Pregnancy and postpartum. Obstetrics & Gynecology Clinics of North America. 2009;36:301-16.

Mottola MF, Davenport MH, Brun CR, Inglis SD, Charlesworth S, Sopper MM. VO2peak prediction and exercise prescription for pregnant women. Medicine & Science in Sports & Exercise. 2006;38(8):1389-95.

Persinger R, Foster C, Gibson M, Fater DC, Porcari JP. Consistency of the talk test for exercise prescription. Medicine & Science in Sports & Exercise. 2004;36(9):1632-6.

Pivarnik, J. Potential Effects of Maternal Physical Activity on Birth Weight: Brief Review. Medicine and Science in Sports and Exercise. 1998; 30(3): 400-6.

Wolfe LA, Mottola MF. Canadian Society for Exercise Physiology [Internet]. Ottawa: Canadian Society for Exercise Physiology. Physical Activity Readiness Medical Examination for Pregnancy. c1999;[last modified 2013; cited Aug 2009]; [about 4 pages]. Available from: http://www.csep.ca/cmfiles/publications/parq/parmed-xpreg.pdf

Chapter 8: Cross Training Your Way Through Pregnancy

ACOG Committee on Obstetric Practice [Internet]. Washington: The American Congress of Obstetricians and Gynecologists. Number 267 Exercise during pregnancy and the postpartum period. c2002; [last modified unknown; cited August 2009]; [about 1 page]. Available from: http://www.acog.org/Resources-And-Publications/Committee-Opinions/Committee-on-Obstetric-Practice/Exercise-During-Pregnancy-and-the-Postpartum-Period.

Artal R, O'Toole M. Guidelines of the American College of Obstetricians and Gynecologists for exercise during pregnancy and the postpartum period. British Journal of Sports Medicine. 2003;37(1):6-12.

Clapp, JF III. Exercising through your pregnancy. Omaha: Atticus Books; 2002.

Davies GA, Wolfe LA, Mottola MF, MacKinnon C. Joint SOGC/CSEP clinical practice guideline: exercise in pregnancy and the postpartum period. Canadian Journal of Applied Physiology, 2003;28(3):330-41.

Moore KL, Dalley AF. Clinically oriented anatomy, fourth edition. Philadelphia: Lippincot, Williams & Wilkins; 1999.

Wolfe LA, Mottola MF. Canadian Society for Exercise Physiology [Internet]. Ottawa: Canadian Society for Exercise Physiology. Physical Activity Readiness Medical Examination for Pregnancy. c1999; [last modified 2013; cited Aug 2009]; [about 4 pages]. Available from: http://www.csep.ca/cmfiles/publications/parq/parmed-xpreg.pdf

Chapter 9: Monitoring the Health of You and Your Baby

Alleyne J, Peticca P. Canadian Academy of Sport and Exercise Medicine [Internet]. Ottawa: Canadian Academy of Sport and Exercise Medicine. Exercise and Pregnancy Position Statement and Discussion Paper; c2008 [last modified unknown; cited August 2009]; [about 18 pages]. Available from: http://casem-acmse.org/wp-content/uploads/2013/07/Discussion-Paper-Pregnancy.pdf

Clapp, JF III. Exercising through your pregnancy. Omaha: Atticus Books; 2002.

Hale RW, Milne L. The elite athlete and exercise in pregnancy. Seminars in Perinatology. 1996;29(4):277-84.

Chapter 10: Getting Sidelined

Alleyne J, Peticca P. Canadian Academy of Sport and Exercise Medicine [Internet]. Ottawa: Canadian Academy of Sport and Exercise Medicine. Exercise and Pregnancy Position Statement and Discussion Paper; c2008 [last modified unknown; cited August 2009]; [about 18 pages]. Available from: http://casem-acmse.org/wp-content/uploads/2013/07/Discussion-Paper-Pregnancy.pdf

Hutchinson A. How your iron levels affect your athletic performance. The Globe and Main [Internet]. Toronto: c2013 Jun 9 [2013 Jul 5; cited 2013 Nov]. Available from: http://www.theglobeandmail.com/life/health-and-fitness/fitness/piecing-together-the-complex-links-between-iron-levels-and-exercise/article12419294/

Malmqvist S, Kjaermann I, Andersen K, Okland I, Bronnick K, Larsen J. Prevalence of low back and pelvic pain during pregnancy in a Norwegian population. Journal of Manipulative and Physiological Therapeutics. 2012;35(4):272-8.

Mogren IM, Pohjanen AI. Low back pain and pelvic pain during pregnancy: Prevalence and risk factors. Spine. 2005;30(8): 983-991.

Pivarnik JM, Chambliss HO, Clapp JF, Dugan SA, Hatch MC, Lovelady CA, Mottola MF, Williams MA. Impact of physical activity during pregnancy and postpartum on chronic disease risk. Special communications consensus statement. Medicine & Science in Sports & Exercise. 2006;38:989-1006.

Stuge B, Veierod MB, Laerum R, Vollestad N. The efficacy of a treatment programs focusing on specific stabilizing exercises for pelvic girdle pain after pregnancy. A two year follow-up of a randomized clinical trial. Spine. 2004;29(10); E197-E203.

Vladutiu CJ, Evenson KR, Marshall SW. Physical activity and injuries during pregnancy. Journal of Physical Activity & Health. 2010;76(6):761-9.

Vleeming A, Albert HB, Ostgaard HC, Stureson B, Stuge B. European guidelines for the diagnosis and treatment of pelvic pain. European Spine Journal. 2008;17:794-819.

Vullo VJ, Richardson JK, Hurvitz, EA. Hip, knee, and foot pain during pregnancy and the postpartum period. Journal of Family Practice. 1996;43(1):63-8.

Pennick V, Liddle SD. Interventions for preventing and treating pelvic and back pain in pregnancy. Cochrane Database of Systematic Reviews. 2013 Aug 1;8:CD001139. doi: 10.1002/14651858.CD001139.pub3.

Chapter 11: Fuelling Your Pregnant Body
Ainsworth BE, Haskell WL, Jermann SD, Meckes N, Bassett DR Jr, Tudor-Locke C, et al. Compendium of physical activities: A second update of codes and MET values. Medicine & Science in Sports & Exercise. 2011;43:1575-81.

Health Canada [Internet]. Ottawa: Health Canada. My Food Guide Servings Tracker; c2011 [last modified 2011 Nov 08; cited 02 Feb 2014]; [about 1 screen]. http://www.hc-sc.gc.ca/fn-an/food-guide-aliment/track-suivi/table_female-femme_preg-ence_age19-50-eng.php

Mayo Clinic Staff [Internet]. Exercise for weight loss. Rochester: Mayo Foundation for Medical Education and Research. c1998-2014 [cited Jan 2014]; [about 1 screen]. Available from: http://www.mayoclinic.org/healthy-living/weight-loss/in-depth/exercise/art-20050999

Chapter 12: Preparing for the Big Event
Alleyne J, Peticca P. Canadian Academy of Sport and Exercise Medicine [Internet]. Ottawa: Canadian Academy of Sport and Exercise Medicine. Exercise and Pregnancy Position Statement and Discussion Paper; c2008 [last modified unknown; cited August 2009]; [about 18 pages]. Available from: http://casem-acmse.org/wp-content/uploads/2013/07/Discussion-Paper-Pregnancy.pdf

Clapp, JF III. Exercising through your pregnancy. Omaha: Atticus Books; 2002.

The American College of Obstetricians and Gynecologists Committee on Obstetric Practice Society for Maternal-Fetal Medicine [Internet]. Washington: The American Congress of Obstetricians and Gynecologists. Committee Opinion No. 579. Definition of term pregnancy. American College of Obstetricians and Gynecologists; cNov 2014; [last modified unknown; cited August 2014]. Available from: http://www.acog.org/Resources-And-Publications/Committee-Opinions/Committee-on-Obstetric-Practice/Definition-of-Term-Pregnancy

Domenjoz I, Kayser B, Boulvain M. Effect of physical activity during pregnancy on mode of delivery. American Journal of Obstetrics and Gynecology. 2014;211:401.e1-11.

Mayo Clinic Staff [Internet]. Stages of labor: Baby its time! Rochester: Mayo Foundation for Medical Education and Research. c1998-2014 [cited Jan 2014]; [about 2 screens]. Available from: http://www.mayoclinic.org/healthy-living/labor-and-delivery/in-depth/stages-of-labor/art-20046545

Singata M, Tranmer J, Gyte GML. Restricting oral fluid and food intake during labour. Cochrane Database of Systematic Reviews 2013, Issue 8. Art. No.: CD003930. DOI: 10.1002/14651858.CD003930.pub3.

Cunningham GF, Whitridge WJ, Leveno KJ, Bloom SL, Hauth JC, Rouse DJ, et al. Williams Obstetrics. 23rd ed. New York: McGraw Hill; 2009.

GETTING YOUR GROOVE BACK

Chapter 13: A Holistic Approach to Getting Your Groove Back
Albright CL, Maddock JE, Nigg CR. Physical activity before pregnancy and following childbirth in a multiethnic sample of healthy women in Hawaii. Women and Health. 2005;42:95-110.

Alleyne J, Peticca P. Canadian Academy of Sport and Exercise Medicine [Internet]. Ottawa: Canadian Academy of Sport and Exercise Medicine. Exercise and Pregnancy Position Statement and Discussion Paper; c2008 [last modified unknown; cited August 2009]; [about 18 pages]. Available from: http://casem-acmse.org/wp-content/uploads/2013/07/Discussion-Paper-Pregnancy.pdf

Brumitt J. A return to running program for the postpartum client: A case report. Physiotherapy Theory and Practice. 2009;25(4):310-25.

No Authors. Impact of physical activity during pregnancy and postpartum on chronic disease risk. Medicine & Science in Sports & Exercise. 2006;38(5):989-1006.

Reimer LJ. The postpartum challenge. Get fit with a program designed for you and your baby. American Fitness, 2007;25(3):58-61.

Chapter 14: Respecting Your New Body
Al-Sayegh NA, George SE, Boninger ML, Rogers JC, Whitney SL, Delitto A. Spinal mobilization of postpartum low back and pelvic girdle pain: An evidence-based clinical rule for predicting responders and nonresponders. Physical Medicine and Rehabilitation. 2010;2:995-1005.

Bo K, Backe-Hansen KL. Do elite athletes experience low back, pelvic girdle and pelvic floor complaints during and after pregnancy? Scandinavian Journal of Medicine & Science in Sports. 2007;17:480-7.

Clapp, JF III. Exercising through your pregnancy. Omaha: Atticus Books; 2002.

Dube R. Marathon moms raise the post-natal bar. Toronto: Globe and Mail [Internet]. c2006 Nov. [last modified 2012 Aug 22; cited Feb 2008]. Available from: http://www.theglobeandmail.com/life/parenting/marathon-moms-raise-the-post-natal-bar/article4266077/

Jefferys R. The pregnant exerciser: An argument for exercise as a means to support pregnancy. ACSM's Certified News. 2005;15(3):5-7.

Memon HU, Handa VL. Vaginal childbirth and pelvic floor disorders. Women's Health. 2013;9(3):265-77.

Press Association. Paula Radcliffe plans gentle return to racing after childbirth. UK: The Guardian [Internet]. c2010 [last modified unknow; cited May 2011]. Available from: http://www.theguardian.com/sport/2010/jun/11/paula-radcliffe-return-childbirth

Stone CA. Visceral and obstetric osteopathy. Edinburgh: Churchill Livingstone Elsiever; 2007.

Stuge B, Veierod MB, Laerum R, Vollestad N. The efficacy of a treatment programs focusing on specific stabilizing exercises for pelvic girdle pain after pregnancy. A two year follow-up of a randomized clinical trial. Spine. 2004;29(10);E197-E203.

Vleeming A, Albert HB, Ostgaard HC, Sturesson B, Stuge B. European guidelines for the diagnosis and treatment of pelvic girdle pain. European Spine Journal. 2008;17:794-819.

Pivarnik JM, Chambliss HO, Clapp JF, Dugan SA, Hatch MC, Lovelady CA, Mottola MF, Williams MA. Impact of physical activity during pregnancy and postpartum on chronic disease risk. Special communications consensus statement. Medicine & Science in Sports & Exercise. 2006;38:989-1006.

Chapter 15: Phase 1: Your Initial Recovery

Kawaguchi JK and Pickering RK. The pregnant athlete, part 3: Exercise in the postpartum period and return to play. Athletic Therapy Today. 2010;15(4):36-41.

Williams A, Herron-Marx S, Carolyn H. The prevalence of enduring postnatal perineal morbidity and its relationship to perineal trauma. Midwifery. 2007;23(4):392-403.

Wolfe LA, Mottola MF. Canadian Society for Exercise Physiology [Internet]. Ottawa: Canadian Society for Exercise Physiology. Physical Activity Readiness Medical Examination for Pregnancy. c1999;[last modified 2013; cited Aug 2009]; [about 4 pages]. Available from: http://www.csep.ca/cmfiles/publications/parq/parmed-xpreg.pdf

Chapter 16: Phase 2: Your Ongoing Recovery and Light Exercise

Clapp, JF III. Exercising through your pregnancy. Omaha: Atticus Books; 2002.

Kawaguchi JK and Pickering RK. The pregnant athlete, part 3: Exercise in the postpartum period and return to play. Athletic Therapy Today. 2010;15(4):36-41.

Reimer LJ. The postpartum challenge. Get fit with a program designed for you and your baby. American Fitness. 2007;25(3):58-61.

Chapter 17: Phase 3: Your Structured Training Program

Kawaguchi JK and Pickering RK. The pregnant athlete, part 3: Exercise in the postpartum period and return to play. Athletic Therapy Today. 2010;15(4):36-41.

O'Mara K [Internet]. San Diego: Competitor Group Inc. Can women come back faster after pregnancy? c2013 October 3 [last modified 2014 May 10; cited February 2014]. Available from: http://running.competitor.com/2013/10/training/can-women-come-back-faster -after-pregnancy_61244

Reddy L, Gheerbrant J. [Internet]. London: BBC Sport Athletics. Jessica Ennis-Hill: Could pregnancy make her better? c2014[last modified January 2014; cited February 2014]. Available from: http://www.bbc.com/sport/0/athletics/25680341

Chapter 18: The Breastfeeding Athlete

Alleyne J, Peticca P. Canadian Academy of Sport and Exercise Medicine [Internet]. Ottawa: Canadian Academy of Sport and Exercise Medicine. Exercise and Pregnancy Position Statement and Discussion Paper; c2008 [last modified unknown; cited August 2009]; [about 18 pages]. Available from: http://casem-acmse.org/wp-content/uploads/2013/07/Discussion-Paper-Pregnancy.pdf

Artero EG, Ortega FB, Espana-Romero V, Labayen I, Huybrechts I, Papadaki A, et al. Longer breastfeeding is associated with increased lower body explosive strength during adolescence. Journal of Nutrition. 2010;140 (11):1989-95.

Carey GB, Quinn TJ, Goodwin SE. Breast milk composition after exercise of different intensities. Journal of Human Lactation. 1997;13(2):115-20.

Clapp, JF III. Exercising through your pregnancy. Omaha: Atticus Books; 2002.

Daley AJ, Thomas A, Cooper H, Fitzpatrick J, McDonald C, Moore H, et al. Maternal exercise and growth in breastfed infants: a meta-analysis of randomized control trials. Pediatrics. 2012;130(1):108-14.

Dewey, KG. Effects of maternal caloric restriction and exercise during lactation. The Journal of Nutrition. 1998;128(2 Suppl):386S-389S.

Dewey KG, Lovelady CA, Nommsen-Rivers LA, McCrory MA, Lonnerdal B. A randomized study of the effects of aerobic exercise by lactating women on breast-milk volume and composition. New England Journal of Medicine. 1994;330(7):449-53.

Health Canada [Internet]. Ottawa: Health Canada. Infant Feeding; c2012 [last modified 2014 May 27; cited 05 Jan 2014]; [about 1 screen]. Available from: http://www.hc-sc.gc.ca/fn-an/ nutrition/infant-nourisson/index-eng.php

Hrysomallis C. Effectiveness of strengthening and stretching exercises for the postural correction of abducted scapulae: A review. Journal of strength and Conditioning Research. 2010;24(2):567-74.

Lovelady CA, Lonnerdal B, Dewey KG Lactation performance of exercising women. The American Journal of Clinical Nutrition. 1990;52(1):103-9.

Lovelady CA, Hunter CP, Geigerman C. Effect of exercise on immunologic factors in breast milk. Pediatrics. 2003;111(2):E148-52.

Lovelady CA, Bopp MJ, Colleran HL, Mackie HK, Wideman. Effects of exercise training on loss of bone mineral density during lactation. Medicine & Science in Sports & Exercise. 2009;41(10):1902-7.

Wood LA, Wade K, Fordham J, Mather J, Jovkovic O. Breastfeeding in Toronto. Promoting supportive environments. Toronto Public Health. March 2010.

Wright KS, Quinn TJ, Carey GB. Infant acceptance of breast milk after maternal exercise. Pediatrics. 2002;109(4):585-9.

Young M. [Internet]. EliteTrack Sport Training & Conditioning. A review on postural realignment and its muscular and neural components; c2008 [last modified unknown; cited August 2014]; [about 11 pages]. Available from: http://www.elitetrack.com/article_files/posture.pdf

GOING THE EXTRA MILE

Chapter 19: Expanding Your Support Team

American Pregnancy Association [Internet]. Texas: American Pregnancy Association. Chiropractic care during pregnancy; c2012 April 27 [last modified 2014 Jan; cited June 2014]; [about 1 screen]. Available from: http://americanpregnancy.org/pregnancy-health/chiropractic-care-during-pregnancy/

Canadian Association of Naturopathic Doctors [homepage on the Internet]. Toronto: The Canadian Association of Naturopathic Doctors; c1999-2014 [last updated unknown; cited 2014 June]. Available from: https://www.cand.ca

Canadian Chiropractic Association [homepage on the Internet]. Toronto: The Canadian Chiropractic Association; c2014 [last update unknown; cited 2014 June]. Available from: http://www.chiropractic.ca

Canadian Physiotherapy Association [homepage on the Internet]. Ottawa: The Canadian Physiotherapy Association; c2012 [last updated 2014; cited 2014 June]. Available from: http://www.physiotherapy.ca/Home

Field T, Hernandex-Reif M, Taylor S, Quintino O, Burman I. Labor pain is reduced by massage therapy. Journal of Psychosomatic Obstetrics and Gynaecology. 1997;18(4):286-91.

Field T, Hernandez-Reif M, Hart S, Theakston H, Schanberg S, Kuhn C. Pregnant women benefit from massage therapy. Journal of Psychosomatic Obstetrics and Gynaecology. 1999;20(1):31-8.

Hollenbach D, Broker R, Herlehy S, Stube K. Non-pharmacological interventions for sleep quality and insomnia during pregnancy: A systematic review. The Journal of the Canadian Chiropractic Association. 2013;57(3):260-70.

Jefferys R. The pregnant exerciser: An argument for exercise as a means to support pregnancy. ACSM's Certified News. 2005;15(3):5-7.

Lavelle JM. Osteopathic manipulative treatment in pregnant women. The Journal of the American Osteopathic Association. 2012;112(6):343-6.

Licciardone JC, Buchanan S, Hensel KL, King HH, Fulda KG, Stoll ST. Osteopathic manipulative treatment of back pain and related symptoms during pregnancy: A randomized control trial. American Journal of Obstetrics and Gynecology. 2010;202(1):43e1-43e8.

Ontario Association of Manual Practitioners [homepage on the Internet]. Toronto: The Association of Manual Practitioners; c2014 [cited 2014 June]. Available from: http://osteopathyontario.org

Pennick V, Liddle SD. Interventions for preventing and treating pelvic and back pain in pregnancy. Cochrane Database of Systematic Reviews. 2013 Aug 1;8:CD001139. doi: 10.1002/14651858.CD001139.pub3.

Smith CA, Levett KM, Collins CT, Jones L. Massage, reflexology and other manual methods for pain management in labour (Review). The Cochrane Database of Systematic Reviews, 2012, Issue 2. Art. No.: CD009290. DOI: 10.1002/14651858.CD009290.pub2.

Stuber KJ, Wynd S, Weis CA. Adverse; events from spinal manipulation in the pregnant and postpartum periods: a critical review of the literature. Chiropractic & Manual Therapies. 2012;20:8. http://chiromt.com/content/20/1/8

Steel A, Adams J, Sibbritt D, Broom A, Gallois C, Frawley J. Utilisation of complementary and alternative medicine (CAM) practitioners within maternity care provisions: results from a nationally representative cohort study of 1,835 pregnant women. BMC Pregnancy and Childbirth. 2012;12:146.

Vermani E, Mittal R, Weeks A. Pelvic girdle pain and low back pain in pregnancy: A review. Pain Practice. 2010;10(1):60-71.

Vleeming A, Albert HB, Ostgaard HC, Sturesson B, Stuge B. European guidelines for the diagnosis and treatment of pelvic girdle pain. European Spine Journal. 2008;17:794-819.

Walker J. The effect of Osteopathic treatment during pregnancy on the outcomes of labour and delivery [Internet]. 2007 [updated 2011; cited May 2014]. Available from: http://www. torontoosteopathy.com/About-Me.aspx

Yuen T, Wells K, Benoit S, Yohanathan S, Capelletti L, Stuber K. Therapeutic interventions employed by Greater Toronto Area chiropractors on pregnant patients: results of a cross-sectional online survey. The Journal of the Canadian Chiropractic Association. 2013;57(2):132-42.

Chapter 20: Your Strong and Powerful Core

Benjamin DR, van de Water ATM, Peiris CL. Effects of exercise on diastasis of the rectus abdominis muscle in the antenatal and postnatal periods: a systematic review. Physiotherapy. 2014;100(1):1-8.

Bewyer KJ, Bewyer DC, Messenger D, Kennedy CM. Pilot data: Association between gluteus medius weakness and low back pain during pregnancy. The Iowa Orthopaedic Journal. 2009;29:97-9.

Brumitt J. A return to running program for the postpartum client: A case report. Physiotherapy Theory and Practice. 2009; 25(4):310-25.

Coldron Y, Stokes MJ, Newham DJ, Cook K. Postpartum characteristics of rectus abdominis on ultrasound imaging. Manual Therapy. 2008;13:112-21.

Gutke A, Ostgaard HC, Oberg B. Association between muscle function and low back pain in relation to pregnancy. Journal of Rehabilitation Medicine. 2008;40:304-11.

Teyhen DS, editor. JOSPT Perspectives for Patients. Pregnancy and low back pain. Physical therapy can reduce back and pelvic pain during and after pregnancy. Journal of Orthopaedic & Sports Physical Therapy. 2014;44(7):474.

Moore KL, Dalley AF. Clinically oriented anatomy, fourth edition. Philadelphia: Lippincot, Williams & Wilkins; 1999.

Tupler J. Maternal Fitness: Preparing for a health pregnancy, an easier labor, and a quick recovery. New York: Fireside, 2006.

McGill S. Low back disorders: Evidence-based prevention and rehabilitation. Human Kinetics Publishers, 2007.

Rajalakshmi D, Kumar NSS. Strengthening transversus abdominis in pregnancy related pelvic pain: The pressure biofeedback stabilization training. Global Journal of Health Science. 2012;4(4):55-61.

Jennifer Faraone & Dr. Carol Ann Weis

Thein-Nissenbaum JM, Thompson EF, Chumanov ES, Heiderscheit B. Low back and hip pain in a postpartum runner: Applying ultrasound imaging and running analysis. Journal of Orthopaedic & Sports Physical Therapy. 2012;42(7):615-24.

van Benten E, Pool J, Mens J, Pool-Goudzwaard A. Recommendations for physical therapist on the treatment of lumbopelvic pain during pregnancy: A systematic review. Journal of Orthopaedic & Sports Physical Therapy. 2014;44(7):464-71.

University Health Services [Internet]. New Jersey: Princeton University. Lumbar/core strength and stability exercises. c2011 [last modified 2011;cited 2014 May 2014]; [about 3 screens]. Available from: https://www.princeton.edu/uhs/pdfs/Lumbar.pdf

Weis CA, Nash J, Triano JJ, Barett J. Abdominal muscle thickness and low back pain during pregnancy; A preliminary study. Proceedings of the Association of Chiropractic College-Research Agenda Conference (Abstract). Journal of Chiropractic Education. 2011;25(1):p75.

Weis CA, Triano JJ, Barrett J, Campbell MD, Croy M, Roeder J. Abdominal thickness in postpartum versus nulliparous women: A preliminary study. Proceedings of the Association of Chiropractic College-Research Agenda Conference (Abstract). Journal of Chiropractic Education. 2009;23(1):p100.

Chapter 21: Your Silent Training Partner - Your Pelvic Floor Muscles

Bernardes BT, Resende AP, Stupp L, Oliveira E, Castro RA, Bella ZI, Girao MJ, Satori MG. Efficacy of pelvic floor muscle training and hypopressive exercises for treating pelvic organ prolapse in women: randomized controlled trial. Sao Paulo Medical Journal. 2012; 130(1):5-9.

Berzuk K. I laughed so hard I peed my pants!: A woman's essential guide for improved bladder control. Winnipeg: Incontinence & Pelvic Pain Clinic; 2003.

Bo K, Backe-Hansen KL. Do elite athletes experience low back, pelvic girdle and pelvic floor complaints during and after pregnancy? Scandinavian Journal of Medicine & Science in Sports. 2007;17:480-7.

Boyle R Hay-Smith EJV, Cody JD, Morkved S. Pelvic floor muscle training for prevention and treatment of urinary and faecal incontinence in antenatal and postnatal women (Review). Cochrane Database Systematic Review. 2012, Issue 10. Art. No.: CD007471. DOI: 10.1002/14651858.CD007471.pub2.

The Canadian Continence Foundation [homepage on the Internet]. Peterborough: The Canadian Continence Foundation. c2014 [cited May 2014]. Available at: http://www.canadiancontinence.ca/EN/index.php

Dumoulin C, Hay-Smith J. Pelvic floor muscle training versus no treatment, or inactive control treatments, for urinary incontinence in women. Cochrane Database Systematic Review. 2014, Issue 5. Art. No.: CD005654. DOI: 10.1002/14651858.CD005654.pub3.

312

Henderson JW, Wang S, Egger MJ, Masters M, Nygaard I. Can women correctly contract their pelvic floor muscles without formal instruction? Female Pelvic Medicine and Reconstructive Surgery. 2013;19(1):8-12.

Jones KA and Moalli PA. Pathophysiology of pelvic organ prolapse. Female Pelvic Medicine and Reconstructive Surgery. 2010;16(2):79-89.

Knorst MR, Cavazzotto K, Henrique M, Resende TL. Physical therapy intervention in women with urinary incontinence associated with pelvic organ prolapse. Revista Brasileira de Fisioterapia. 2012;16(2):102-7

Kruger JA, Dietz HP, Murphy BA. Pelvic floor function in elite nulliparous athletes. Ultrasound in Obstetrics and Gynecology. 2007;30:81-5.

Moore KL, Dalley AF. Clinically oriented anatomy, fourth edition. Philadelphia: Lippincot, Williams & Wilkins; 1999.

The National Association for Continence [homepage on the Internet]. South Carolina: The National Association for Continence. c2012 [last updated 2012 Oct 3; cited May 2014]. Available from: http://www.nafc.org

Nygaard IE, Rao SS, Dawson JD. Anal incontinence after anal sphincter disruption: a 30-year retrospective cohort study. Obstetrics and Gynecology. 1997;89(6):896-901.

Nygaard I, Barber MD, Burgio KL, Kenton K, Meikle S, Schaffer J, et al. Prevalence of symptomatic pelvic floor disorders in US women. The Journal of the American Medical Association. 2008;300(11):1311-6.

Patel DA, Xu X, Thomason AD, Ransom SB, Ivy JS, DeLancey JD. Childbirth and pelvic floor dysfunction: an epidemiologic approach to the assessment of prevention opportunities at delivery. American Journal of Obstetrics and Gynecology. 2006;195(1):23-8.

Rortveit G, Brown JS, Thom DH, Van Den Eeden SK, Creasman JM, Subak LL Symptomatic pelvic organ prolapse: prevalence and risk factors in a population-based, racially diverse cohort. Obstetrics and Gynecology. 2007;109(6):1396-403.

Stepp, KJ, Walters, MD. Anatomy of the lower urinary tract, rectum and pelvic floor. In: Urogynecology and Reconstructive Surgery, 3rd ed, Walters, M, Karram, M (Eds). Philadelphia: Mosby; 2007. p 24.

Sze EH, Sherard GB 3rd, Dolezal JM. Pregnancy, labor, delivery, and pelvic organ prolapse. Obstetrics and Gynecology. 2002;100(5 pt 1):981-6.

Williams A, Herron-Marx S, Carolyn H. The prevalence of enduring postnatal perineal morbidity and its relationship to perineal trauma. Midwifery. 2007;23(4):392-403.

ABOUT THE AUTHORS

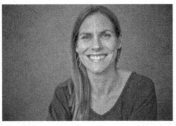

Jennifer Faraone is a competitive athlete, coach, writer and most importantly, a mother. She and her husband have spent the last several years balancing their athletic lifestyle while raising their two young and energetic children. She participates in numerous races, encompassing road running, trail running or duathlons. Her many accomplishments include winning gold and bronze medals at the World Duathlon Championships, a first place finish at the Toronto Half Marathon and representing Canada at the World Mountain Running Championship. But much of her passion with sports lies with helping others to be fit and encouraging them to create an active lifestyle that works for them and their family. She coaches other athletes in the Toronto area, hosts trail running clinics and camps and writes for several fitness magazines and other sources. She can be contacted at jennifer.faraone@yahoo.ca or www.runningthetrails.wordpress.com.

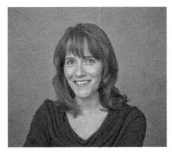

Dr. Carol-Ann Weis is a chiropractor at 2 multidisciplinary clinics in Toronto and has worked in the health and fitness industry for over 20 years. She graduated from the University of Western Ontario with a Bachelor of Arts (Honours) in Physical Education and a Master of Science in Exercise Physiology, where she specifically looked at exercise during pregnancy. Several years later, she graduated from the Canadian Memorial Chiropractic College. Carol Ann has since combined the knowledge and experience from both her careers in order to meld the disciplines of fitness and chiropractic, providing the utmost care to her patients. She has worked with all types of patients, from the weekend warrior to the elite athlete and from children to the elderly. Carol Ann continues to work in the fitness industry as a personal trainer, as well as lectures and conducts research on back pain and pregnancy at CMCC. She presents her research at a number of conferences and has co-authored two manuals for fitness certifying bodies, as well as a variety of articles for the fitness industry. Carol Ann is an avid cyclist and runner, was a member of the National Duathlon Team and qualified twice for the World Duathlon championship. She can be contacted at drcarolannweis@gmail.com.

Printed in the United States
By Bookmasters